The New Medical School Preparation & Admissions Guide

5th Edition

NEW & UPDATED FOR TOMORROW'S MEDICAL SCHOOL APPLICANTS AND PREMED STUDENTS

Dr. Andrew Goliszek

Healthnet Press

Southport, NC

Library of Congress Catalog Card Number: 2024912937

Dr. Andrew Goliszek

The New Medical School Preparation & Admissions Guide

ISBN: 978-0-9616475-7-5

Healthnet Press

Contents

Also by Andrew Goliszek

Nonfiction

How Anyone Can Learn Anything

Stress, Disease and the Mind-Body Connection

Mind-Body Health & Self-Healing

In the Name of Science: A History of Human Experimentation

60-Second Stress Management

Breaking the Stress Habit

The Complete Medical School Preparation & Admissions Guide

Fiction

Rivers of the Black Moon

World Order

Like Embers in the Night

Acronyms and Abbreviations

The most used acronyms and abbreviations used by premedical and medical students are provided here for your convenience.

AAMC: Association of American Medical Colleges

ABMS: American Board of Medical Specialties

AMA: American Medical Association

AMCAS: American Medical College Application Service

DAT: Dental Admission Test

DO: Doctor of Osteopathic Medicine (Osteopathic Physician)

EDP: Early Decision Program

FAFSA: Free Application for Federal Student Aid

FAP: Fee Assistance Program

FOAM: Free Open Access Medical Education

FSMB: Federation of State Medical Boards

HBCU: Historically Black Colleges and Universities

LCME: Liaison Committee on Medical Education

MCAT: Medical College Admission Test

MD: Doctor of Medicine (Allopathic Physician)

MED-MAR: Medical Minority Application Registry

NBME: Board of Medical Examiners

NRMP: National Residency Matching Program

OAT: Optometry Admission Test

PCAT: Pharmacy College Admission Test

PGY: Post Graduate Year

SMDEP: Summer Medical and Dental Education Program

TMDAS: Texas Medical and Dental Schools Application

USMLE: United States Medical Licensing Examination

VCAT: Veterinary College Admission Test

WICHE: Western Interstate Commission for Higher Education

WWAMI: Washington, Wyoming, Alaska, Montana, and Idaho

INTRODUCTION

If you're deciding or have already decided on a career in medicine, you're most likely a good student, you enjoy science, you're motivated and ambitious, and you have a strong desire to do something worthwhile with your life. You may have thought about being a physician while in high school and are now ready to take the steps necessary to make it a reality. Because so many students choose medicine as a career, your chances for admission will improve considerably if you begin a systematic plan of action that will get you ready for that final decision. By starting now, you'll avoid many of the problems and pitfalls that face so many students.

Every year, more than one million college freshman register either as premed majors or have plans to take courses that will qualify them to apply to one of the nation's 155 accredited M.D. or 37 accredited D.O. programs. By their senior year, only about 60,000 take the MCAT, and in 2023-24, only about 23,000 got accepted to medical school. Applications over the last few year have increased, partly because the COVID pandemic has inspired some applicants to seek careers in medicine. What the rejections don't show, however, is that grades and MCAT scores are not enough, and that other factors can make or break a student's chances of success. The key to successful admission is knowing the specific qualities medical schools are looking for and then beginning a strategy that will boost the odds that you'll be one of the lucky few that get accepted.

Before doing anything else, you must do a self-analysis. Be honest with yourself when answering the following questions because your answers are important in helping you decide if medicine is the right career path for you.

Why do I want to be a doctor?

Am I pursuing medicine because it's expected of me?

Am I going into medicine mainly for financial reasons?

Do I have a sense of compassion for others?

Am I honest and trustworthy?

Am I willing to work long hours and make sacrifices to be a medical student?

Am I willing to be around sick and dying people?

Do I have the desire and fortitude to put up with sometimes intolerable conditions?

Do I have excellent communication skills?

Am I a team player and work well with others?

Am I intelligent enough to absorb an incredible amount of information?

Do I consider myself a lifelong learner?

Many of the questions deal with personality traits of successful students, and personal qualities a physician must have in his or her dealings with patients and colleagues. If you're not ready or able to spend countless hours studying or are not inquisitive enough to constantly search for answers to questions, then medicine is not for you. Likewise, if you're not willing to be part of a team, which is the trend in medical education, or are not thorough, diligent, self-disciplined, and conscientious, getting through medical school will be next to impossible. Only you can decide if you have the personal qualities essential to get you through four exceedingly difficult years.

If you've answered the questions honestly and still believe you have what it takes to be a good candidate, you need to begin preparing as soon as possible. Too many students procrastinate, neglect their studies, ignore non-academic factors medical schools look for, and miss important deadlines. In the chapters ahead, I'll discuss new trends in medical school education and in admission policies, and offer a wealth of information that will increase your chances for success.

CHAPTER 1

MEDICAL SCHOOL EDUCATION

Medical curricula and teaching philosophies are similar among medical schools, but just as universities differ in how they approach teaching, medical schools also differ in how they structure coursework, electives, and rotations. However, because all medical students must take national boards to get licensed, every program is consistent in its goal of preparing students for graduation. In light of that, one of the major changes affecting new medical students is the emphasis on reasoning and critical thinking skills, and the ability of candidates not only to absorb and understand complex material but also to interpret and analyze that material in order to make informed decisions. Doctors of the future will also need to be more team-oriented, where decisions are based on consensus and teamwork.

This change is reflected in the new version of the entrance exam, the MCAT, which includes a greater emphasis on reasoning, critical thinking, and problem-solving skills. The purpose of the new format, which went into effect in 2015, is to make sure that potential medical students are not simply memorizers of information but are better able to think through and analyze information and make informed decisions. The following statement, made by a professor of medical pharmacology at the medical school I was affiliated with, expresses his view of what a medical education is all about:

"I think of medical school more like an advanced trade school than a university. Students come here to learn a specific trade and must know certain facts to qualify to perform that trade. Our purpose is not so much to dwell on theoretical aspects of medicine but rather to give students the tools needed to become physicians. But to be a physician, one needs to acquire an incredible amount of information and facts, and to be able to use that information and those facts intelligently and critically to make life or death decisions. An important part of medical training is teaching students how to think."

Pathway to Becoming a Physician

Your journey from undergraduate student to physician, especially if you want to become a specialist, is long and arduous. It takes patience, diligence, motivation, determination and, above all, a lot of hard work and long hours of study. A medical student once told me that if you took everything you learned in your college science classes and multiplied it by a thousand, that would be medical school. Here's a simplified flowchart that describes the steps along the way:

4-Year College or University
(B.S. or B.A. with the required coursework)

↓

4-Year Medical School (M.D. or D.O. degree)

↓

3-6 Year Residency Training

↓

1-3 Year Optional Fellowship in a Subspecialty

Depending on your interests and career goals, expect to spend anywhere from 8 to 13 years after graduating from college to finally being a practicing physician. During that time, there will be an internship, a residency, and an optional fellowship, if you choose to subspecialize in a specialty. There will also be medical board exams after your second year of medical school, and then again during your fourth year and after your first year of residency. To become board certified in a specialty, there's a comprehensive examination at the end of the residency period.

Because of the incredible amount of material presented, medical students learn early on how to study efficiently, how to be good time managers, and how to be team players. They form great study habits, and they cooperate with classmates to get through the stress and the rigors of medical school. According to medical school educators, the most successful students are the ones who possess these five qualities:

- Strong motivation and discipline.
- Ability to pursue problems in great depth.
- A capacity for sustained scholarship.
- Critical thinking skills.
- A persistent sense of desire to seek answers to problems.

Having these qualities doesn't necessarily mean that an individual will get through four years of medical school with flying colors. Not having them, however, can mean a great deal of trouble in keeping up with classmates you'll be competing against for choice spots in limited residency programs. So before thinking about a career in medicine, consider whether you're willing to make the enormous sacrifices needed to be successful every step of the way.

The Affordable Care Act and Medical Education

According to the American Medical Association, the Affordable Care Act (ACA) has not only changed the landscape of healthcare, but it will influence how medical students approach their education and the choices they make after graduation. The demand for physicians is projected to grow by almost 20 percent because of the ACA, with demand significantly exceeding supply. Total shortages by 2025, based on AAMC findings, will be between 12,500 and 31,100 primary care physicians and between 28,200 and 63,700 non-primary care physicians. This truly is a good time to consider a career in medicine.

Two major provisions of immediate relevance to medical students are their education debt and what they do after their residencies. Here are the major provisions of the ACA as they relate to future doctors:

- The ACA improves the National Health Service Corps (NHSC) Loan Repayment Program. In the provision, the repayment amount is increased from $35,000 to $50,000 for the initial 2-year service requirement. It also increases funding to address physician shortages in high need areas and allows part-time service and teaching to qualify towards the NHSC service requirement.
- Students who qualify for loan forgiveness through NHSC will no longer have to count that as taxable income when submitting their federal income tax as physicians.
- The ACA provides $1.5 billion to the NHSC to recruit and train primary care physicians and surgeons to work in rural and underserved areas. It also increases incentives to go into primary care by providing a 10% bonus and increased Medicaid payments for primary care physicians.
- By redistributing the number of Medicare-funded training positions in areas where they are needed most, students may not be able to get the residencies they apply for.

In addition to the provisions of the ACA, prospective medical students will need to familiarize themselves with other new changes in healthcare because all these changes are going to have a profound impact on the schools they choose, the residencies they apply for, and the way they practice medicine for the rest of their lives. Students who dream of becoming specialists for financial reasons, for example, are going to be disappointed that salaries are not going to be as high as they once were. And students who think that specialties are the wave of the future will be surprised to learn that primary care is really the future of medicine.

A study that followed 2,500 medical students over a period of twenty years found that 30 percent of those who entered medical school wanting to be primary care physicians changed their minds and chose a higher-paying specialty. The main reason was debt and worries about paying back student loans. What graduates will discover by the end of the decade is that a 5-year residency is not necessarily going to pay off because the environment will have completely changed, and the big salaries will not be there any longer.

The other major trend caused by the ACA is that fewer doctors will be working for themselves in private practice and, instead, will be joining large groups or becoming employees of hospitals and insurance companies. "Everything seems to be changing, and I have no idea what to do anymore," said a premedical student I talked to recently. This student, like so many others, needs to become familiar with the law and the changes, and plan accordingly. To find out more about the Affordable Care Act, visit www.hhs.gov /healthcare. To learn more about the National Health Service Corps and how it will impact you as a student, visit their site at www.nhsc.hrsa.gov.

M.D. versus D.O. Degree

Allopathic physicians (M.D.s) and osteopathic physicians (D.O.s) both complete four years of medical school, are held to the same standards, choose the same residency programs in order to practice in any medical specialty, and take similar tests for board certification. The main difference is that osteopathic physicians receive additional training in hands-on manual medicine and the body's musculoskeletal system.

Osteopathic medicine concentrates on treating and healing the whole person rather than focusing on an individual organ system or diseased body part. Because of this approach, D.O.s will often use a technique called osteopathic manipulative treatment or OMT to make sure that the body is moving freely, and body fluids are flowing normally. For example, while an M.D. may diagnose and treat a headache with medication, a D.O. may also include manipulation of the neck and spine, much like a chiropractor would.

Experience causes the osteopathic physician to develop a highly sensitive touch that allows him or her to literary feel the patient's anatomy. Not all D.O.s use OMT; and the vast majority use many of the surgical techniques used by medical doctors. So when deciding on an M.D. versus a D.O. degree, it's personal preference. Students who want to focus on treating the whole patient and ensuring that all the body's natural healing systems are working together may want to consider osteopathic medicine as a career.

Students choosing the D.O. path may also want to consider attending an osteopathic residency program rather than an allopathic residency program. The specialty you choose can make a difference in which residency program best suits you and where you'll find the best training to meet your needs. So before applying, do some research, make some contacts, and decide which type of program will enhance your future career goals.

Personality Traits of Successful Medical Students

One of the new trends in medical school admissions is examining personality traits of applicants, in addition to considering more cognitive factors such as GPA and MCAT. Because medical school is so difficult, and because schools invest so much time and effort in training physicians, it is becoming increasingly important to predict which type of student will be most successful. According to studies, there are certain personality traits that medical schools are looking for because these traits have been shown to be good predictors of success. They are:

- **Self-discipline and competence:** The first two years of a medical school program has a strong emphasis on science courses. The very rigorous curriculum can take a toll on students if they're not motivated and self-disciplined, not to mention extremely competent in study, learning, and test-taking skills. Before any other trait is considered, medical schools must determine that an applicant has the self-discipline to get through four tough years and the unusually high intelligence required to absorb the amount of material necessary to become a physician.
- **Conscientiousness:** Following two years of science courses, students will transition to clinical experiences, where interpersonal skills such as dependability and attention to detail are especially important. For students to succeed, they not only need to be conscientious, but also honest, agreeable, and have a genuine concern for the wellbeing of others. They also need to have a genuine interest in what they're doing.
- **Interpersonal skills:** During the first two years of medical school, students will depend on each other for support and cooperation in preparing for courses and studying for exams. They cannot be afraid to ask for help if they need it. The last two years are the clinical years, where interpersonal skills and team effort are critical. Students who do not cooperate, who are not agreeable, and who do not work as a team are not going to be successful in clerkships and residencies.
- **Emotional stability:** It goes without saying that getting through medical school requires a lot of sacrifices, and there will be times when students get depressed and feel as if they cannot handle the pressure. Being emotionally strong and having a good support system is essential for success. One of the things admissions interviewers look for is whether they feel the applicant has the emotional fortitude to make it through their program.
- **Time Management Skills:** If there's one constant in medical school, it's stress. If a student cannot cope with stress because of procrastination or poor time management skills, he or she will have a difficult time getting things done, may get physically ill, and will find it impossible to stay on track. The most successful students are the ones who thrive in stressful situations because they know how to handle pressure and have learned to manage their time well.

No single personality type makes the best doctor, but lacking certain traits will make it that much more difficult to successfully complete an M.D. degree. Prospective applicants need to take a step back and consider whether they have the personality and the motivation it takes to become a physician. If they do, then medicine may very well be the perfect career choice.

Variety in Medical School Programs

In general, the time needed to complete the requirements for an M.D. degree is four years. However, there are some accelerated programs that allow graduation in less time, which I'll discuss later in the book. Each school accredited by the Association of American Medical Colleges has curricula that are similar, although electives can vary, as can the order of classes, the number and types of required courses, and the time sequence in which students would take those courses. Therefore, what seems attractive to one applicant may not be the right fit for another. Prospective students need to look at each school's catalogue for the most recent changes and additions and see how different schools train their doctors in their own unique way.

Regardless of time allotted to coursework, and the differences in academic systems, the nature of the curricula is basically the same. During the first two years, students focus on basic sciences that include anatomy, biochemistry, physiology, cell and molecular biology, genetics, histology, pharmacology, and behavioral science, among other topics. These subjects are often presented in modules of several weeks to several months in length. Again, the order of subjects and the manner in which they're presented may vary from school to school. Some schools prefer to integrate courses and to inter-relate them with the organ systems. Other schools take an independent approach and teach the courses separately.

Over the next decade, medical school programs and the way they're designed will be more flexible. Some schools, rather than expecting students to spend their first two years sitting in a classroom and reading textbooks, are requiring them to start working with patients while they learn basic sciences. Others are building facilities that focus on interdisciplinary team-based instruction where students learn in small groups. The design of the future is a school loaded with technology, spaces that mimic emergency rooms containing full-body simulation mannequins for hands-on training, and flexible classrooms for smaller groups of students that can interact and problem-solve.

Whatever the approach, the aim of a medical school curricula is to prepare medical students for (1) step 1 of the United States Medical Licensing Exam, which is taken after the second year of study, (2) the final two years of clinical medicine, which emphasize the application of basic sciences to the solution of clinical problems and the practice of medicine, and (3) the residency years, in which students put into practice what they've been taught. While schools may differ in their philosophies and in how they approach their teaching, the high pass rates on medical licensure exams indicate that all schools do a remarkable job of preparing their students to become successful physicians.

Examples of Medical School Curricula

A visit to any medical school website will give you an idea of what each school year is like, and the kinds of courses and clerkships required for graduation. The following four examples are actual curricula from four different medical schools. The first two are private schools and are either highly or less competitive; the last two are public and are either highly or less competitive. They illustrate the similarities and differences in a four-year medical education regardless of whether a school is private or is more competitive than another.

The first two years are typically filled with science coursework and medical-related topics. The last two years focus on clerkships that last anywhere from 2 to 12 weeks, advanced electives, and internships in various specialties. One of the factors to think about when selecting potential medical schools is how their curricula will enhance your education and your future as a physician. Consider this carefully because it can really influence not only your success but your ability to land the residency or fellowship of your choice.

School A: Private, Highly Competitive

1st Year	Molecular and Cell Physiology, Metabolism and Endocrinology, Molecular and Human Genetics, Sexual Development and Reproduction, Special Senses, Medical Neuroscience, Clinical Ethics, Ambulatory Care, Physical Diagnosis
2nd Year	Immune Regulation, Hematology, Virology, Bacteriology and Mycology, Cardiovascular, Renal and Genitourinary, Upper Respiratory and Pulmonary, Physical Diagnosis, Neurologic Disorders, Psychiatric Disorders, Health Care Ethics, Gastrointestinal and Hepatic, Endocrine, Orthopedic, Rheumatology, Dermatology, Pediatrics, Geriatrics
3rd Year	*Clerkships*: Family Medicine, Internal Medicine, Neurology, Obstetrics and Gynecology, Pediatrics, Psychiatry, General Surgery, Surgical Specialties
4th Year	Internships in various specialties and subspecialties, Electives

School B: Private, Less Competitive

1st Year	Principles of Medicine, Introduction to Disease, Neuroscience, Health Care Ethics, Medical Humanities, Clinical Skills, Evidence Based Medicine I, Palliative Care I, Professionalism I, System Based Practice I
2nd Year	Hematology, Oncology, Cardiovascular, Respiratory, Renal and Genitourinary, Gastrointestinal and Nutrition, Endocrinology, Reproduction, Human Sexuality, Evidence Based Medicine II, Palliative Care II, Professionalism II, System Based Practice II
3rd Year	*Clerkships*: Family Medicine, Internal Medicine, Neurology, Obstetrics and Gynecology, Pediatrics, Psychiatry, General Surgery, Surgical Specialties
4th Year	Alcohol and Drug Dependence Treatment, ICU, Emergency Medicine, Acting Internships, 24 weeks of Elective Rotations

School C: Public, Highly Competitive

1st Year	Molecular and Cell Biology, Structure and Development, Integrative Function, Microbial Pathogens, Clinical Skills Development, Medicine and Society

2nd Year — Hematology, Oncology, Cardiovascular, Respiratory, Gastrointestinal, Urinary and Renal, Brain and Behavior, Endocrine and Nutrition, Reproductive Medicine, Genetics, Musculoskeletal, Dermatology, Diagnosis and Therapy, Clinical Skills, Humanities and Social Sciences, Clinical Epidemiology

3rd Year — *Clerkships*: Family Medicine, Inpatient Medicine, Neurology, Obstetrics and Gynecology, Pediatrics, Psychiatry, Surgery, Intro to Acute Care

4th Year — Advanced Practice, Acting Internship, Critical Care, Science of Medicine, Electives, Capstone Course

School D: Public, Less Competitive

1st Year — Behavioral Sciences, Doctoring I, Ethics and Social Issues in Medicine I, Anatomy and Embryology, Medical Biochemistry, Medical Histology, Microbiology and Immunology I, Neuroscience, Medical Physiology, Primary Care Medicine

2nd Year — Doctoring II, Ethics and Social Issues in Medicine II, Intro to Medicine, Medical Genetics, Medical Microbiology and Immunology II, Pathology, Pharmacology, Psychopathology, Primary Care

3rd Year — *Clerkships*: Family Medicine, Internal Medicine, Obstetrics and Gynecology, Pediatrics, Psychiatric Medicine, Surgery, Cardiovascular Care, Radiology, Clinical Elective Rotation

4th Year — Community-Based Primary Care, Acting Internship, ICU, Emergency Medicine, Clinical Neuroscience, 14 Weeks of Electives, Capstone

Clinical Clerkships

After the first two years of a basic science curriculum, students begin a year of clerkships in which they put their knowledge and skills to work with real patients in hospitals and other clinical settings. It's during this year that they learn the fundamentals of physical examination, evaluation, diagnosis, and patient care in various specialties. It's also a time when medical students begin to think about further study in one of those specialties or subspecialties.

During clerkships, students rotate every few weeks or months through different medical departments and interact with patients under the supervision of senior attending physicians. Schools may differ slightly in the type and length of clerkships required, but in general they're similar in that students receive critical hands-on experience in a real-life hospital setting. Depending on the medical school, clerkships last anywhere from 15 to 18 months and include a core clinical requirement. Students may also have to choose an elective clerkship, a clinical care clerkship, and a pre-internship clerkship as part of an M.D. degree.

Subinternships

A Subinternship, sometimes referred to as an acting internship or AI, is a fourth-year clinical rotation at a hospital other than the one in which the medical student is affiliated. After completing the 3rd year clerkships, students will often select certain subinternships because of career interest. During the AI, a student will perform the role of an intern under the supervision of a senior attending physician. Common Subinternships are Internal Medicine, Surgery, and Pediatrics. If a medical student is planning to apply for residency at a specific institution, he or she will often select that institution to do a subinternship to gain an advantage when eventually applying.

Medical schools will often use subinternships to prepare fourth-year students for the internship, which can be a demanding and rigorous experience. The goal is to expand on what students have learned during clerkship rotations, and to enhance skills needed to treat and manage patients, all under the supervision of senior physicians.

Internships

The first year of training after a student has graduated from medical school is called an internship or PGY-1 (Post Graduate Year-1). This is the first year of residency, when the intern begins making rounds with a team of other interns, a supervising resident, and an attending physician. During this first year, interns rotate through various specialties or subspecialties before settling on their own specialty.

Students who want to become general practitioners perform a one-year internship before getting licensed. These one-year internships are flexible and designed to provide a wide range of clinical experiences. Duties include attending lectures and seminars, ordering and analyzing labs, performing medical procedures, and, of course, preparing for medical licensure exams. Those who decide on a specialty will spend an additional 3 to 5 years as a resident (see the list of specialties and subspecialties later in the chapter).

Residency

The term residency refers to a 3 to 5-year training program in a medical specialty following the internship (PGY-2, PGY-3, etc.). Because this is the time to learn just about everything you'll need to know about your specific field, the more time you spend and the more patients you see, the more proficient you'll become as a specialist. If you choose surgery, practice makes perfect, so as a surgical resident you'll spend much of your time helping perform surgeries.

A typical day starts early, often at 7AM, and includes rounds to visit patients, take histories, do physical exams, check lab results, oversee therapy, and discuss care. Residents also attend conferences and lectures to enhance their knowledge base and keep up with the latest medical information. After hours, a resident may check in with his or her patients again or spend time studying. The more hands-on experience a resident gets, the more he or she can help pass on that experience in what is referred to as "see one, do one, teach one." The first time you observe, the next few times you do the procedure, and then, once you become proficient, you teach someone else to do it.

While in residency, students are periodically scheduled to stay at a hospital overnight to care for patients and new admissions. This may require a resident to work up to 36 hours and is a long-standing tradition in medicine. The reason for this, according to medical educators, is that the more hours and experience you get in treating patients, the better a doctor you will become. As you progress from one year to the next, you'll gain valuable knowledge and experience and will do less of the menial and grunt work, which is reserved for first year interns.

The American Medical Association lists the various residencies, along with the number of slots available, when to apply and interview, and the salaries for each year of residence. Because residents are not fully licensed to practice medicine, they're paid a minimum salary of about $50,000 to $70,000 depending on the institution. These "physicians in training" work under the supervision of attending physicians responsible for the patients and are the ones generating revenue for the medical facility.

Students may also choose between university-based residency programs versus community-based residencies depending on their career goals and where they would ultimately like to practice medicine. For example, if your goal is to work at a prestigious medical institution or in a large metropolitan area, it would be to your advantage to do your residency at a university-based program. If your goal is to work in a smaller community or at a small local hospital, then it wouldn't matter where you choose to do your residency.

Once a medical student chooses several programs of interest, he or she will go through a selection process, which includes an interview and a ranking of the top choices by both the applicant and the program. The programs then rank their top candidates, and matches are made to determine which candidates will be selected to which programs. These matches are made by the National Resident Matching Program (NRMP), a non-profit corporation that feeds the information from every medical student into a computer and then matches students and residency programs with their highest preferences.

On match day, which is usually on the same day in mid-March, the selections are revealed, and the applicants find out where they will be training for the next several years. Once students are matched, they're committed to accept that program. If a student does not get matched into a residency program, he or she can participate in what's called the Scramble, a way to get unmatched students into unfilled positions for which they're eligible. During the past few years, the number of unfilled residency positions has decreased, especially in certain specialties. According to the NRMP, orthopedic surgery had only 4 open spots for 142 applicants while family medicine had 153 open spots but only 29 applicants. And with healthcare changes coming, there may be more dramatic decreases in the number of specialty positions available. To learn more about the Match Program, visit *www.nrmp.org.*

Residency Trends

According to the National Resident Matching Program, the 2023 residency match was the largest in NRMP history with more than 48,000 registered applicants vying for just over 40,000 certified residency positions. The AAMC predicts that because the U.S. will face a shortage of as many as 90,000 doctors, residency positions will continue to expand, with key growth in primary care. As many as 52,000 primary care physicians will be needed by 2025.

With new medical schools either being established or in the planning stages, and with increasing medical school enrollments, the number of seniors and the number of positions offered is at an all-time high. That statistic is likely to continue. When we dig into the numbers, we can see some residency trends:

- More than half of new first-year positions were in the primary care specialties of Family Medicine, Internal Medicine, Emergency Medicine, and Pediatrics. 95 percent of Family Medicine programs were filled, 99 percent of Internal Medicine programs were filled, and almost 100 percent of Pediatrics programs were filled.
- Sixty percent of the growth in first-year positions is attributed to primary care, with internal medicine having the biggest increase among all primary care specialties.
- The overall match rate was 75% with 52% of graduates matched to their first choice.
- Some of the most competitive specialties that offered at least 20 first-year positions and were 100 percent filled were: Dermatology, Psychiatry, Obstetrics and Gynecology, Orthopedic Surgery, Pediatrics-Primary Care, Physical Medicine/Rehabilitation, and Thoracic Surgery. General Surgery, Neurological Surgery, Otolaryngology, Plastic Surgery, and Radiation Oncology had fewer than 5 unfilled positions.
- The number of graduates from U.S. medical schools is expected to surpass the number of positions in residency programs. In 2023, almost 10,000 graduates (25%) did not get matched. Since preference is given to U.S. seniors, it will be almost impossible for international medical graduates to get into residency programs.

Fellowships

Any advanced training done in a subspecialty following a residency is called a fellowship. Some medical specialties require one or more years of fellowship training in addition to the three to five years of residency. Fellows, as they're called, act as attending physicians in the field they're trained and, once they've completed their fellowship, can practice in their chosen field without supervision by other physicians.

Several programs offer combined fellowships, in which the fellow trains in two or more subspecialties. As an example, pulmonary/critical care or hematology/oncology are two such combined subspecialties. The list of specialties and subspecialties later in the chapter includes the typical length of a fellowship in a medical field of study.

Primary Care and the Future of Medical Education

A primary care physician is someone you see first for checkups and for any undiagnosed health problems. After completing four years of medical school with an M.D., graduates planning on becoming primary care physicians take postgraduate training in internal medicine, pediatrics, or family medicine, which take a minimum of three additional years of residence. One of the main reasons most medical students choose specialties like surgery, orthopedics, or neurology rather than become primary care physicians is the huge disparity in incomes. But by the end of this decade, a shift in healthcare will change everything we've come to expect from our healthcare system.

The way in which the U.S. system is structured today is that primary care physicians refer patients to specialists who, in turn, take over the care of the patient and who are associated with a specific hospital. In the near future, healthcare will be centered on the primary care physician, while specialists and hospitals will become partners in caring for the sick patient. This team approach is what's going to level the salary playing field and make primary care physicians the leaders in healthcare delivery. Besides, with an increasing patient base and a decreasing number of students choosing primary care, the law of supply and demand will assure that those entering primary care will be rewarded for their work.

Although most graduates choose a field other than primary care, some schools are gradually seeing an increase. At the University of Hawaii, for example, 50 percent of the 2020 graduating class chose primary care, one of the highest percentages of students choosing primary care in the nation. One of the main factors in attracting students is the curricula, which emphasizes preventative and alternative medicine. As more schools try these kinds of innovative approaches, and as the Affordable Care Act places a premium on prevention and health management, more and more students will opt for primary care as their medical career of choice. If you're interested in a career as a primary care physician and want to be at the forefront of a changing healthcare system, look for medical schools with programs designed for that purpose.

How FOAM Will Change Medical Education

FOAM is the acronym for **Free Open Access Medical Education**, an expanding database that includes online videos, iTunes lectures, podcasts, modules, tweets, and blogs that encourage study and active learning. In essence, it's a new way of instantly sharing medical resources so that students and physicians can keep up with evolving technology, techniques, and the latest information. It's the perfect transition to a system that will use the electronic devices students have grown up with and are intimately familiar with.

Because FOAM is personalized and continually expanding, sometimes by the hour, students supplement textbooks containing information that may be outdated, with devices that have internet capability. For example, students can be anywhere and decide to pull up information on a cell phone or an iPad instead of flipping through a 1,200-page textbook. Or within minutes, they can be watching a podcast with a lecture on the latest procedure or cancer treatment. The simplicity of FOAM allows anyone to access resources without having to be in a lecture hall or classroom. And the best part is that most of these resources are free.

The reason medical schools are embracing FOAM is that it enhances learning by encouraging medical students to participate actively in discussions. By nature, medical students are inquisitive and driven to pursue knowledge. They're also life-long learners who never stop searching for answers to their questions. FOAM is the perfect solution for a student who needs to watch a 15-minute video or read about the latest developments in breast cancer. But the main reason medical schools will rely more and more on FOAM is that, as the adage goes, "you can't diagnose what you don't know." By using this new technology, students will learn more, know more, become more engaged, and graduate as much better doctors.

Fields of Specialty and Subspecialty

Starting in their first year, medical students are often asked, "What specialty are you thinking about?" Most students have some idea what they might be interested in, but many do not. Determining a specialty is probably the most important step in a student's career, and it depends on several factors. Some students care more about work schedules and flexibility than they do about income. Others may find life balance and family life more important than the stress of working in a high-profile field.

Personality also plays a key role. Students have to decide if they would rather work behind the scenes or spend more time interacting with people, or whether they prefer being in a hospital setting much of their day or in an office consulting with their patients. Whatever the choice, it is always a difficult and very personal decision.

Most medical school graduates choose a field of specialty or subspecialty during their third or fourth year. A few go on to Ph.D. programs if they wish to develop careers as medical scientists, and some go back later to residency programs. The following is a list of specialties and subspecialties that graduates choose once they have completed a four-year medical degree. There may be some differences in residency length from state to state, but in general the time required for board certification is the same.

Allergy & Immunology: Diagnosis and treatment of various allergies such as asthma, hay fever, etc., and diseases associated with the immune system.

Subspecialty: None
Residence length: 3 years.
Projected increase through 2025: -10%
Further information: www.aaaai.org

Anesthesiology: Administration of anesthesia prior to and during surgery.

Subspecialties: Adult Cardiac anesthesiology, Critical Care Medicine, Hospice and Palliative Medicine, Pain Management, Pediatric Anesthesiology, Sleep Medicine
Residence length: 4 years

Fellowship length: 1 year
Projected increase through 2025: 23%
Further information: www.painmed.org

Colon and Rectal Surgery: Diagnosis, treatment, and surgical management of diseases of the colon and rectum.

Subspecialties: None
Residence length: 5 years
Projected increase through 2025: 22%
Further information: www.fascrs.org

Dermatology: Diagnosis and treatment of skin disorders and diseases.

Subspecialties: Dermatopathology, Pediatric Dermatology
Residence length: 4 years
Fellowship length: 1 year
Projected increase through 2025: 16%
Further information: www.aad.org

Emergency Medicine: Treatment and surgical management of emergency cases such as accidents, traumas, and immediate life-threatening situations.

Subspecialties: Anesthesiology Critical Care Medicine, Emergency Medical Services, Hospice and Palliative Care, Internal Medicine Critical Care, Medical Toxicology, Pain Medicine, Pediatric Emergency Medicine, Sports Medicine, Undersea and Hyperbaric Medicine
Residence length: 3-4 years
Fellowship length: 1-2 years
Projected increase through 2025: 29%
Further information: www.acep.org

Family Medicine: Diagnosis and treatment of diseases and illnesses of all family members and the general health care of adults and children within the family unit.

Subspecialties: Adolescent Medicine, Geriatric Medicine, Hospice and Palliative Care, Pain Medicine, Sleep Medicine, Sports Medicine
Residence length: 3 years
Fellowship length: 1 year
Projected increase through 2025: 21%
Further information: www.aafp.org

Internal Medicine: Diagnosis and treatment of adult internal disorders.

Subspecialties: Adolescent Medicine, Cardiovascular Disease, Clinical Cardiac Electrophysiology, Critical Care Medicine, Endocrinology, Diabetes and Metabolism, Gastroenterology, Geriatric Medicine, Hematology, Hospice and Palliative Medicine, Infectious Disease, Interventional Cardiology, Nephrology, Oncology, Pulmonary Disease,

Rheumatology, Sleep Medicine, Sports Medicine, Transplant Hepatology
Residence length: 3 years
Fellowship length: 1-3 years
Projected increase through 2025: 21%
Further information: www.acponline.org

Medical Genetics: Diagnosis and treatment of genetic-based illnesses and disorders. First two years are completed in another specialty such as pediatrics or internal medicine.

Subspecialties: Clinical Biochemical Genetics, Clinical Cytogenetics, Clinical Genetics, Clinical Molecular Genetics, Medical Biochemical Genetics, Molecular Genetic Pathology
Residence length: 4 years
Fellowship length: 1 year
Projected increase through 2025: 13%
Further information: www.acmg.net

Neurological Surgery: Diagnosis, treatment, and surgical management of the brain, spinal cord, and nervous system.

Subspecialties: None
Residence length 7 years
Fellowship length: 1-2 years
Projected increase through 2025: 4%
Further information: www.neurosurgery.org

Neurology: Diagnosis and treatment of nervous system disorders, as well as certain muscle disorders and pain problems.

Subspecialties: Brain Injury Medicine, Child Neurology, Clinical Neurophysiology, Epilepsy, Neuromuscular Medicine, Pain Medicine, Vascular Neurology
Residence length: 4 years
Fellowship length: 1 year
Projected increase through 2025: 23%
Further information: www.aan.com

Nuclear Medicine: Use of radioactive materials for diagnostic treatment. Administering radionuclides intravenously to scan brain, skeleton, liver, bone marrow, etc. for tumors, diseases, and other abnormalities.

Subspecialties: None
Residence length: 4 years
Projected increase through 2025: 8%
Further information: www.snm.org

Obstetrics and Gynecology: Care and treatment of pregnancy and childbirth, or care and treatment of female disorders.

Subspecialties: Critical Care Medicine, Female Pelvic Medicine and Reconstructive Surgery,

Gynecologic Oncology, Hospice and Palliative Medicine, Maternal and Fetal Medicine, Reproductive Endocrinology/Infertility
Residence length: 4 years
Projected increase through 2025: 18%
Further information: www.acog.org

Ophthalmology: Care and treatment of eye disorders

Subspecialties: None
Residence length: 4 years
Fellowship length: 2 years
Projected increase through 2025: 2%
Further information: www.eyenet.org

Orthopedic Surgery: Diagnosis, treatment, and surgical management of bone, joint, muscle, cartilage, and ligament.

Subspecialties: Orthopedic Sports Medicine, Surgery of the Hand
Residence length: 5 years
Fellowship length: 1 year
Projected increase through 2025: 3%
Further information: www.aaos.org

Otolaryngology: Diagnosis, treatment, and surgical management of disorders of all head cavities.

Subspecialties: Complex Pediatric Otolaryngology, Neurotology, Pediatric otolaryngology, Plastic Surgery within the Head and Neck, Sleep Medicine
Residence length: 5 years
Fellowship length: 2 years
Projected increase through 2025: 3%
Further information: www.entnet.org

Pathology: Study and identification of the causes of disease.

Subspecialties: Blood Banking/Transfusion Medicine, Clinical Informatics, Cytopathology, Dermatopathology, Neuropathology, Chemical Pathology, Forensic Pathology, Hematology, Medical Microbiology, Molecular Genetic Pathology, Pediatric Pathology
Residence length: 4 years
Fellowship length: 1-2 years
Projected increase through 2025: 6%
Further information: www.cap.org

Pediatrics: Care and treatment of all aspects of childhood disorders and diseases.

Subspecialties: Adolescent Medicine, Child Abuse Pediatrics, Developmental-Behavioral Pediatrics, Hospice and Palliative Medicine, Medical Toxicology, Neonatal-Perinatal Medicine, Neurodevelopmental Disabilities, Pediatric Cardiology, Pediatric Critical Care

Medicine, Pediatric Emergency Medicine, Pediatric Endocrinology, Pediatric Gastroenterology, Pediatric Hematology-Oncology, Pediatric Infectious Diseases, Pediatric Nephrology, Pediatric Pulmonology, Pediatric Rheumatology, Pediatric Transplant Hepatology, Sleep Medicine, Sports Medicine
Residence length: 3 years
Fellowship length: 1-3 years
Projected increase through 2025: 21%
Further information: www.aap.org

Physical Medicine and Rehabilitation: Care, treatment, and restoration of diseased, injured, and defective limbs and other body parts.

Subspecialties: Brain Injury Medicine, Hospice and Palliative Medicine, Neuromuscular Medicine, Pain Medicine, Pediatric Rehabilitation Medicine, Spinal Cord Injury Medicine, Sports Medicine
Residence length: 4 years
Fellowship length: 1 year
Projected increase through 2025: 38%
Further information: www.aapmr.org

Plastic Surgery: Surgical management that involves the appearance of any body part.

Subspecialties: Plastic Surgery within the Head and Neck, Surgery of the Hand
Residence length: 6 years
Fellowship length: 1 year
Projected increase through 2025: -4%
Further information: www.plasticsurgery.org

Preventive Medicine: Specializing in the prevention of diseases within the community, the environment, and industry.

Subspecialties: Aerospace Medicine, Clinical Informatics, Toxicology, Occupational Medicine, Public Health and General Preventive Medicine, Undersea and Hyperbaric Medicine
Residence length: 3 years
Fellowship length: 1-2 years
Projected increase through 2025: -11%
Further information: www.asma.org

Psychiatry: Care and treatment of behavioral and emotional disorders.

Subspecialties: Addiction Psychiatry, Child and Adolescent Psychiatry, Forensic Psychiatry, Geriatric Psychiatry, Hospice and Palliative Care, Neurodevelopmental Disabilities, Psychosomatic Medicine, Sleep Medicine
Residence length: 4 years
Fellowship length: 1-2 years
Projected increase through 2025: 11%

Further information: www.psych.org

Radiology: Use of X-rays to diagnose physical disorders for the purpose of medical treatment.

Subspecialties: Diagnostic Radiology, Radiation Oncology, Medical Physics, Neuroradiology, Nuclear Radiology, Pediatric Radiology, Vascular and Interventional Radiology
Residence length: 5 years
Fellowship length: 1 year
Projected increase through 2025: 1%
Further information: www.acr.org

Surgery, General: Surgical management of any part of the body.

Subspecialties: Complex General Surgical Oncology, Pediatric Surgery, Surgery of the Hand, Surgical Critical Care, Vascular Surgery
Residence length: 5 years
Fellowship length: 1-2 years
Projected increase through 2025: 18%
Further information: www.facs.org

Thoracic Surgery: Surgery involving organs of the chest.

Subspecialties: Congenital Cardiac Surgery
Residence length: 6 years
Fellowship length: 1 year
Projected increase through 2025: -13%
Further information: www.sts.org

Urology: Diagnosis, management, and treatment of the male urogenital and female urinary tract. The first year must be in general surgery.

Subspecialties: Female Pelvic Medicine and Reconstructive Surgery, Pediatric Urology, Neurourology, Renal Transplantation
Residence length: 5 years
Fellowship length: 1 year
Projected increase through 2025: -7%
Further information: www.auanet.org

Top 10 In-Demand Medical Specialties

Despite the emphasis on primary care over the next decade, there will always be a demand for specialists. According to the Department of Health and Human Services, certain specialties will remain the same or decline, as will the number of residency positions, while the demand for certain medical specialists will increase.

Because of an aging population and changes in healthcare, some specialties will increase dramatically over the next 10-20 years. The following are the top ten specialties that are projected to grow the fastest:

1. Family Medicine
2. Psychiatry
3. Internal Medicine
4. Emergency Medicine
5. Child and Adolescent Psychiatry
6. Obstetrics and Gynecology
7. Anesthesiology
8. Urgent Care
9. Geriatric Medicine
10. Hematology/Oncology

Choosing a Medical Specialty

Most first-year students have at least some idea of what they'd like to specialize in after they graduate. Some don't have a clue because they've not been exposed enough to different fields of medicine to know. In general, medical students choose a specialty based on several factors:

1. Their background and personality type and how well their personality fits the lifestyle of the specialty.
2. Their background and their interests.
3. Their natural abilities and talents.
4. Where they would like to live.
5. Whether they would like to do research in their field of specialty.
6. How much time they are willing to spend in the office seeing patients or in a hospital setting.
7. How many years they'll have to spend in a residency program.
8. How much compensation they will get in the specialty.

Sometimes an individual would like to do it all: seeing patients, teaching, and doing research at a teaching hospital. A good way to match a particular specialty with your abilities, interests, values, and personality is to take the Specialty Quiz on the Student Doctor Network at http://schools.studentdoctor.net/selector. Completing the quiz won't tell you which specialty you should pursue, but it will give you an idea of how you match up, given your answers.

When doctors were asked how they finally decided on their specialty, many of them said they made their choices based mainly on their experiences in clinical rotations. Sometimes medical students think they might be interested in a particular specialty until they experience it firsthand. Another common answer was the amount of time they would spend in either an office or a hospital or clinical setting. The following is a chart of the most common specialties and how they compare in terms of time allocated between office and hospital settings.

Time Spent in Office Versus Hospital

Office	Office/Hospital	Hospital/Office	Hospital
⟵			⟶
Dermatology Medical Genetics Preventive Medicine Rheumatology	Allergy & Immunology Cardiology Endocrinology Family Practice Gastroenterology Internal Medicine Nephrology Pediatrics Psychiatry Pulmonary Medicine	Colon/Rectal Surgery General Surgery Hematology Infectious Diseases Medical Oncology Neurological Surgery Obstetrics & Gynecology Ophthalmology Orthopedic Surgery Pediatric Subspecialties Plastic Surgery Thoracic Surgery Urology	Anesthesiology Emergency Medicine Nuclear Medicine Pathology Physical Medicine & Rehabilitation Radiation Oncology Diagnostic Radiology

In some cases, medical students choose specialties early on in their education. But in general, choosing a specialty turns out to be a difficult, personal, and confusing decision.

In fact, as many as seventy five percent of all medical students change their specialty after being exposed to clinical rotations and internships. The best way to make more informed and concrete choices is to follow progressive decision-making rules beginning in the first year of medical school. These are:

First year students: begin thinking about specialties and prepare to make some choices.

Second year students: learn as much as you can about the different specialties and subspecialties, and consider your own interests, abilities, and personality.

Third year students: link your interests and abilities to certain fields of medicine, and then explore those areas in much greater depth. If you find a certain clinical rotation appealing, talk at length to physicians who know the specialty firsthand.

Fourth year students: choose among the few specialties you find equally appealing and try to fit one to your own unique talents as an individual.

The more a student applies this kind of approach, the easier it will be to decide on a particular specialty. For more information regarding the time requirements and details about board certification, go to the American Board of Medical Specialties website at http://www.abms.org.

Emerging Specialties

Some specialties are in greater demand than others. For example, the top five fastest growing specialties during the past five years have been: Family Practice, Sports Medicine Physician, Hospitalist, Emergency Medicine, and Geriatrician. Demand for geriatricians alone will be 30,000 by 2030. There are various other specialty opportunities for doctors that are viewed as "emerging trends" in medicine, some you may never have heard of such as cancer immunologist, nocturnist, lifestyle medicine physician, clinical informatics, and medical virtualist. Medical students interested in these specialties need to know that there aren't as many residency programs or there isn't a sizeable enough group of physicians practicing in that field to have a large number of openings in residency programs. Some may not yet be recognized as official specialties by the American Board of Medical Specialties. Here are some main emerging specialties:

Emerging Specialty	Description / Post-Residency Training
Addiction Medicine	Treatment of patients with alcohol and drug addiction problems. 1-2 years training after a 4-year psychiatry residency.
Administrative Medicine	Management and financial aspects of medical practice. 5-10 years of medical experience in addition to

	business courses.
Adolescent Medicine	A subspecialty of family practice, pediatrics, and internal medicine focuses exclusively on adolescents. 1-3 years after a 3-year residency in family practice, internal medicine, or pediatrics.
Critical Care Medicine	Care of patients with critical illnesses including transportation to the hospital and time in the emergency room. 1-3 years after residency.
Geriatrics	Diagnosis and treatment of the elderly. One year after residency.
Hospice and Palliative Care	Focuses on relieving suffering and controlling symptoms such as pain. One year after residency.
Women's Health	Focuses on women's reproductive health, domestic violence, nutrition, and other issues concerning women. Physicians choosing this practice are typically licensed in OB/GYN, family practice, or psychiatry.

How Much Do Physicians Earn?

According to economic data, going to medical school is the best return on an educational investment there is. Although medical school is expensive, doctors earn a good living, and many graduates receive generous loan repayment offers or low interest rates on existing loans. Salaries vary depending on the region of the country, the state, and the specialty. The following is a 2024 listing of the most common specialties and the average salary that a physician can expect to make after several years of practice. The salaries are listed from the highest to lowest paid specialty and are based on a compilation of several sources that survey doctors nationwide.

Average Physician Compensation

Specialty	Average Salary Range
Plastic Surgery	$476,000 - $676,000
Orthopedics	$457,000 - $657,000
Cardiology	$390,000 - $590,000
Otolaryngology	$369,000 - $569,000
Urology	$361,000 - $561,000

Gastroenterology	$353,000 - $553,000
Dermatology	$338,000 - $538,000
Radiology	$337,000 - $537,000
Ophthalmology	$317,000 - $517,000
Hematology/Oncology	$311,000 - $511,000
Anesthesiology	$305,000 - $505,000
General Surgery	$302,000 - $502,000
Emergency Medicine	$273,000 - $473,000
Critical Care	$269,000 - $469,000
Pulmonary Medicine	$253,000 - $453,000
Obstetrics/Gynecology	$236,000 - $436,000
Pathology	$234,000 - $434,000
Nephrology	$229,000 - $429,000
Neurology	$201,000 - $401,000
Allergy & Immunology	$198,000 - $398,000
Rheumatology	$189,000 - $389,000
Psychiatry	$187,000 - $387,000
Internal Medicine	$164,000 – $364,000
Infectious Diseases	$160,000 - $360,000
Endocrinology	$157,000 - $357,000
Family Medicine	$155,000 - $355,000
Pediatrics	$144,000 - $344,000
Public Health	$143,000 - $343,000

Other factors such as the number of patients seen, number of hours worked, size of the practice, geographic region, and whether the physician is in academics or private practice also determines salary. Some physicians choose lifestyle over work, so while one surgeon can earn $250,000 a year, another may earn three times that. However, there are some trends in medicine that will affect the future compensation of all physicians regardless of specialty. They are:

❑ It's becoming more common for physicians working in hospitals to be paid a base salary plus a bonus, depending on productivity and quality-based outcomes rather than being paid a flat salary.

- ❑ Instead of physicians being expected to be on-call as part of their affiliation with hospitals, they're increasingly being compensated for on-call duties. At some hospitals, for example, specialists such as cardiologists are being compensated a set amount per day for being on-call.

- ❑ Physicians are expected to participate in more administrative duties. Medical directors will be compensated for extra work, and some hospitals are including in their contract compensation for duties above and beyond what the physician normally performs.

- ❑ Small practices are increasingly joining larger groups and hospitals to take advantage of advanced technology and ancillary services that generate more revenue than could be generated by individual practices. The era of small or individual practices is becoming a thing of the past.

- ❑ Government reimbursement rates and managed care rates are changing, so compensation rates for physicians will also change over the next several years. Physicians will always be well compensated for what they do; it just may not be as much as it has been in the past.

Medical Licensing Examination

Each state has its own rules and regulations for medical licensure. Many require only one year of an approved internship following medical school to obtain a license to practice medicine as a general practitioner. Most medical students, however, will choose specialties and will need to also pass board certification exams. In the United States, the pathway to a medical license is straightforward:

- Graduation from a medical school approved by the Liaison Committee on Medical Education (LCME), a joint committee of the American Medical Association (AMA) and the Association of American Medical Colleges (AAMC).
- Passing the United States Medical Licensing Examination (USMLE), a multi-part examination given by the Federation of State Medical Boards (FSMB) and the National Board of Medical Examiners (NBME).
- Letters of reference.
- Review of malpractice history.

The USMLE tests an applicant's ability to apply all the knowledge he or she has acquired during four years of medical school. There are three parts to the test, and all three must be passed before an individual is eligible to apply for an unrestricted medical license. First time pass rates for graduates of U.S. medical schools are typically more than 95 percent. The following are the three parts of the USMLE:

Step 1: an 8-hour exam given after a student's second year of medical school that tests one's ability to apply the concepts of basic science to the practice of medicine. This part, which includes approximately 280 questions divided into seven blocks, covers subjects such as anatomy, biochemistry, behavioral sciences, genetics, microbiology, nutrition, pathology, pharmacology, and physiology. The minimum pass rate is 75-percent, but starting January 2022, step 1 was scored as Pass/Fail. One of the reasons this part is so important is that it's often used as a factor in selecting medical students for residency programs. The higher the score, the better the chances are for successful residency applications. If you talk to medical educators, most will tell you that it is the most important exam a medical student will ever take.

Step 2: usually taken during a medical student's fourth year, part 2 of the USMLE tests one's ability to apply knowledge and understanding of clinical science necessary for patient care. This part is divided into two separate exams. The first is a 9-hour exam consisting of approximately 318 questions, divided into 8 blocks, and includes subjects such as Medicine, Pediatrics, Psychiatry, Obstetrics and Gynecology, and Surgery. The second part is a hands-on examination in which each examinee has 15 minutes to examine and take a patient's medical history, and then 10 minutes to write up the findings, offer a diagnosis, and make a list of tests that would be needed. Part 2 is only offered in five cities across the country: Atlanta, Chicago, Houston, Philadelphia, and Los Angeles.

Step 3: the final exam in the USMLE series tests a medical school graduate's ability to apply medical, biomedical, and clinical knowledge in the unsupervised practice of medicine. This part, which had some new changes beginning in 2014, is typically taken at the end of the first-year residency program and is given over a period of two, eight-hour days. The first day consists of 232 multiple-choice questions divided into 6 blocks. The second day includes 180 multiple-choice questions divided into 6 blocks, and thirteen 10-20-minute clinical case simulations where the examinees treat patients, order medications, and monitor the condition of patient changes.

For many students, studying for licensure and practicing for the exam is an ongoing routine. It can be one of the most difficult and stressful times in a student's education, so continuous preparation is a must. For more information on the exam, sample questions, and ways to prepare, go to the USMLE official website at http://www.usmle.org.

Board Certification

Becoming board certified means that you have completed a residency in a specialty and have passed a comprehensive exam in your field of expertise. Although this is a voluntary process, most physicians choose to become board certified to demonstrate their commitment to continually improve in their specialty and provide better care to their patients. Many boards require recertification every 7-10 years, which ensures that physicians are competent and up to date on their specialty or subspecialty.

The American Board of Medical Specialists (ABMS) is responsible for setting the standards for each medical specialty. The first criterion the board looks at is whether a candidate has a valid license to practice medicine. The second is whether that candidate has completed the appropriate residency requirements. If a physician meets those two basic standards, the board will then evaluate the candidate in written and/or practical board examinations; and if the candidate passes, he or she is given the title of Diplomat of that Board. For requirements and more information, visit the American Board of Medical Specialties at http://www.abms.org.

What the Future Holds

Looking at curricula at different medical schools around the country, we get some clues as to what medical education will look like in the future. For students entering classes in 2025 and beyond, and who have grown up around technology and the new changes in healthcare, medical school will be nothing like it was even five years ago. Here are just some of the innovations and new changes being implemented by some of the leading schools in the nation:

- **A focus on technology:** because today's applicants are much more tech savvy, and since medical advances are happening at breakneck speed, medical students need technology to keep up. New buildings and spaces are being created that simulate high tech operating rooms and emergency rooms so that students can practice in real life settings. It's no longer enough to sit in a library and simply read textbooks and journals. Many schools are supplying students with iPads and implementing iPad-based curriculums, which encourage active learning and enhance participation. The University of California-Irvine School of Medicine, for example, became the first medical school to go completely digital, and in 2010 began a comprehensive, iPad-based curriculum. By 2013, they announced that the first class using this new technology scored 23 percent higher on their national exams than previous classes. Expect to see many more of these types of innovations in the future.
- **Combined primary care degree:** since primary care is where healthcare will be focused in the coming years, more schools will be offering combined degrees so that primary care physicians can also practice in other areas of specialization. Brown University Medical School, for example, is beginning a dual degree in primary care and population health to prepare students for a career in which they can do both.
- **Accelerated M.D. degrees:** schools such as the University of California Davis School of Medicine, Texas Tech University School of Medicine, Louisiana State University School of Medicine, and New York University School of Medicine are offering an accelerated three-year medical degree. Two of the main reasons that medical schools are experimenting with a 3-year degree option is to cut the cost of a medical education and to attract more students to pursue careers in primary care. These fast-track programs are not for everyone, but with projections showing that physician shortages will become worse over the next ten years, more schools are looking to accelerated programs as a way to recruit and graduate students who will commit to

primary care.

- **Problem-Based Learning:** students entering medical school today are expected to have a totally different mindset when it comes to approaching their studies. The last ten years have seen more medical advances and breakthroughs than in the previous hundred years combined. The entire DNA molecule has now been sequenced, which means that we will be able to identify and conceivably prevent, treat, or cure almost every possible disease. The goal of problem-based learning in medicine is to help students enhance their problem-solving and learning skills. By working on real patient cases in small groups, medical students develop communication and collaboration skills, as well as becoming more flexible in how they apply their knowledge.
- **Integrating Research Principles:** medical schools are realizing that with medical advances occurring as such a rapid pace, future physicians need to know and be able to use research principles. To do that, many schools are integrating research principles into the curriculum and involving teams of faculty researchers to help students solve health problems based on real-life cases. For example, at the new Oakland University Beaumont School of Medicine, established in 2011, students get extra financial aid in their fourth year if they participate in a research project of significant merit.
- **Skipping residency programs:** some states such as Missouri are addressing the physician shortage by passing laws that would allow medical school graduates to start treating patients without having to spend an extra 3 to 6 years in a residency program. The Missouri law, for example, would issue a license to someone who has graduated from medical school within the past three years and passed the first two rounds of licensing exams within the last two years. These graduates would provide primary care services in medically underserved areas if they are supervised by another physician. Other states such as Arkansas, Kansas, and Oklahoma are also enacting similar measures or considering the idea to meet physician shortages.

With 159 medical schools and 42 DO or osteopathic medical programs in the United States, and more opening in the future, students have a wider range of options than ever. For over 100 years, medical schools have been training doctors in the same way. But that's beginning to change, and the new trend in medical school is to revamp curricula and programs so they reflect the changing face of healthcare and the changing dynamics of modern-day students. Technology is the rage. Modern buildings and facilities that simulate real-life medical situations are becoming more common. Smaller class sizes emphasize teamwork and collaboration among students. And integrating the curricula with patient care early on is the wave of the future. At no time has medical school education been more exciting and challenging. For young students planning a career in medicine, the next ten years will be an incredible decade of both change and opportunity.

CHAPTER 2

THE HIGH SCHOOL YEARS

Is high school too early to begin planning for a future in medicine? Most medical school admissions officers would say no because good high school preparation lays the groundwork for successful admission to top-choice colleges, and ultimately to medical school. One of the main reasons to start thinking about medical school while still in high school is that admissions policies and criteria are changing, the number of applicants will be increasing, and competition is not going to get any easier. Therefore, students who are planning on medical school need to get serious about their education and extracurricular activities and be more prepared than students were in the past.

Building a Solid Foundation

Because of intense competition, not only for admission to medical school but also to select colleges that increase your chances of getting into medical school, the road typically begins in high school. Students who form good study habits and build impressive credentials before applying to college have an advantage over the thousands of other students who think that college is the time to begin taking their education seriously. The fact is that good students who begin early will have the edge and become top candidates.

From my own experiences in dealing with college freshman, I found it essential that students enter college with good fundamentals and a solid foundation. I've seen too many freshmen start slowly, fall behind, and then try to catch up when it's too late. These were basically good students who never developed the study habits needed to make it through a rigorous college program with the kinds of grades necessary for medical school admission. At my university, the number one reason students drop out of premed is chemistry; and the reason for that is they weren't prepared well enough before entering college.

Any good instructor can predict within the first few weeks of class which students will do well just by talking to them about how they prepare for exams and how they study for class. Invariably, the students who excel are the ones who were good high school students and who brought their study and learning skills to college with them. By their senior year, they are the ones being admitted to medical school.

So, how does one build a solid foundation and become the kind of student any college would want? The first thing you must do is make some hard choices. Would you rather spend time partying and socializing, or would you rather participate in clubs and activities that will enhance your high school credentials and prepare you for college? Do you want to waste summers hanging out in your basement playing video games, or do you want to look for summer programs that will expand your horizons, allow you to travel, and to do volunteer work? These, by the way, aren't mutually exclusive. There are many school activities and summer programs that are fun and involve lots of socializing.

The bottom line is that high school should not only be a time of exploration but also a time to develop into a well-rounded student who is organized, disciplined, motivated, and has developed the study skills needed to become a premed. Here are some suggestions that will help high school students build the kind of foundation that will prepare them for a premed curriculum:

- **Develop good study habits.** Premed curriculums are tough. If you want to do well in college, you need to condition yourself early on and develop the study habits that will get you through the courses needed for admission to medical school. Part of good study is learning to be organized and self-disciplined, skills that are critical if you're going to be successful.
- **Improve communication skills.** Oral and written communication skills are a must if you plan on going to medical school. Physicians spend a lot of time writing and communicating with people, so it's important to demonstrate that you can write well and work closely with people from different backgrounds. Becoming active in student organizations and other school activities will help improve your communication skills.
- **Improve reading skills.** Premed and medical students spend a great deal of time reading. Poor readers are not going to make it through a tough curriculum, so enhance your reading skills by reading different types of material, both fiction and non-fiction. Besides reading your textbooks, pick up a newspaper or an article every day and read it, not just for content but for comprehension. The more you read, the faster a reader you'll be.
- **Improve test-taking skills.** From the moment you enter college to the day you get your M.D., you'll be taking exams. There are SATs, ACTs, MCATs, medical boards, and more. Many students cannot get through a premed program because they're poor test-takers. Even a percentage of medical students flunk out of medical school simply because they have a hard time with exams. Don't ruin your chances for success because of poor test-taking skills. And remember, the higher your scores are on the SAT, the greater the likelihood that you'll be accepted to competitive colleges.
- **Take AP classes.** Admissions officers look favorably on students whose transcripts include AP classes. For one, it shows that you have the aptitude to take tough courses. More importantly it shows that you're motivated and are willing to take harder

classes. A rigorous curriculum that includes biology, chemistry, physics, and math looks great on a college application, especially if you're applying to selective colleges.

- **Gain valuable real-world experiences.** With so many good students applying to
- select colleges, extracurricular activities will make you stand out. Summer programs, volunteer work, shadowing experiences with doctors, organizations, and clubs are just some of the ways you can add real world experiences to your resume.

Building a solid foundation will put you head and shoulders above the competition, especially when it comes to applying to select colleges with good track records of medical school acceptance rates. A solid foundation will also make it much easier to transition from high school to college, which can be a difficult time for students not prepared academically. By starting early, high school students will be a step ahead of their classmates and be rewarded for their hard work.

Precollege Coursework

In a later chapter, I'll discuss required and recommended college courses for medical school admissions. But as a high school student, you need to start preparing now to do well in those courses later. Starting off on the right foot in your freshman year will guarantee that you stay on track and maintain good grades. And by taking certain courses in high school, you'll be better prepared for the tough premedical curriculum to come.

According to admissions committee members, premedical education is not only about science courses. A well-rounded applicant must also take non-science courses that are equally important to medical students. An added benefit to beginning your course prep in high school is that you'll do much better on the SAT and enhance your chances of getting accepted into a select college with a record of success in medical school admissions.

Since most college premed curricula are basically the same – one year of biology, one year of physics, and two years of chemistry – taking biology, physics, and chemistry in high school will help you no matter what college you attend. Furthermore, these courses will help prepare you for other health-related curricula. From personal experience working with college freshman, I can tell you that students with a solid background in these courses, especially if they're AP classes, get much better grades.

Recommended Science Courses

To do well in a premed curriculum, you need a strong background in science and math. It doesn't matter whether you get accepted to a highly selective university or a local junior college, taking rigorous high school courses will help you improve your chances of eventually getting into medical school. When asked what the number one factor was in college admissions, colleges overwhelmingly say that it's a rigorous high school curriculum that includes AP classes. For just about any health career, especially medicine, admissions officers and experts recommend that high school students complete the following:

- **4 years of math, including calculus.** Math courses such as algebra and calculus are helpful whether you choose to major in biology or in business administration. Most medical schools require at least one college calculus course, and some require two. By taking an advanced math class, you will also be better prepared for college chemistry and physics, which involves a lot of math. Moreover, math classes force you to think, and anything that forces you to think will naturally help you in other classes.
- **4 years of science, including biology, chemistry, and physics.** A premed curriculum includes a year of biology, a year of physics, and two years of chemistry. Taking these classes in high school (as well as Anatomy & Physiology) will help prepare you better for the rigors of college levels courses. In addition, taking a high school chemistry and physics course will familiarize you with abstract ideas, get you accustomed to the basic math used, and get you thinking in a way that will give you an advantage when you get to college. Finally, college level chemistry is where most premedical students are weeded out, so the more you prepare for chemistry in high school the better you'll do in college. Almost every student I've known who did well in college chemistry has had chemistry in high school.
- **1-2 years of computer science.** It's virtually impossible to get through life today without knowledge of computers. Students who take a computer science class or two will have the skill set needed for other courses that may involve computer technology. One of the trends in medical education is increased technology, and computers are becoming an important part of medical school curricula.

You don't need to take all AP or honors classes, but to get into a select college you must demonstrate that you were willing to push yourself to the limit with more demanding courses. Colleges are always looking at students' records to see how they compare with other applicants at other schools, so you should take as many advanced classes as you can handle. If your school doesn't offer AP courses, then take the most challenging classes available and excel in them.

One of the questions students always ask is whether it's better to get straight A's in regular classes or C's in more difficult AP classes? Given the choice, it's always better to get the A. Few select colleges will forgive too many C's, no matter how difficult the curriculum. Of course the best scenario is to get A's and B's in AP classes because, when selecting applicants, a college will typically give preference to a student who took tough classes and got a B average over a student who got an A average but never took any hard courses.

Recommended Non-Science Courses

Although your focus should be on science and math, don't neglect the non-science classes. These are important in making you a well-rounded student and a better person in general. The non-science courses especially important for future doctors are:

- **English:** Four years of English will improve reading and comprehension skills and make it easier to get through tough courses later. Writing skills are also essential. Almost every college instructor is going to give exams that require some form of essay writing. I've seen many good students get poor grades simply because they had poor writing skills, which made exams much harder than they really were. Writing skills are critical in a student's overall academic success and, as a college professor for many years, I can tell you that you'll be judged by your ability to communicate. Students who write well will almost certainly make a better impression on their teachers, and it will make taking exams much easier. I can also tell you that students who write well will gain a teacher's respect and get the benefit of the doubt when teachers are grading exam questions.
- **Humanities:** The trend in medical school admissions is to recruit well-rounded students with a broad educational base. The time when medical schools accepted science majors almost exclusively is long gone and, according to recent surveys of admissions officers, humanities subjects need to be put back into medical education to improve the human quality of tomorrow's physician. Subjects like literature, art, and social sciences are now considered important factors in helping improve a student's ability to interact with others and with society. By taking more humanities-based courses, schools will look at you as a more cultured, knowledgeable, and interesting person, and that's exactly what medical schools are looking for as well.
- **Languages:** All high schools offer foreign languages; and taking at least two years of a foreign language will make your college application look much better. As far as medical schools go, their emphasis is on science and math skills, although they do look favorably on applicants who have also demonstrated an interest in other subjects. However, always keep in mind that taking languages for four years will never compensate for making C's in chemistry.

Taking non-science courses like literature, art, music, writing, and language adds to your credentials and will make your application much better. More colleges and medical schools are reevaluating the importance of liberal arts in the development of the total physician and are selecting applicants who show an interest in more than just science.

Non-Academic Activities

High school students are always asking how important extracurricular activities are when applying to colleges. The answer depends on what the rest of the college application looks like. If participating in activities is going to overwhelm you to the point that you have little time to study and your grades suffer, then extracurricular activities can be a negative. However, if you can maintain your grades while being involved in a few good activities, then they can make you stand out.

The number and types of activities you're involved in can also make a difference to an admissions officer. Colleges look for depth, commitment, and leadership, and not just numbers. In fact, participating in five or more extracurricular activities a year is usually a red flag indicating that all you're trying to do is pad your application. That's a big mistake. It's better to do one or two things well and stick with it for the long term than just get involved with something short term to make yourself look good. No one activity is better than another, if you're committed to that activity and demonstrate that you genuinely care about what you're doing. Having a leadership role is a big plus. The following are some examples of high school activities to consider:

- **The Arts:** theater, dance, school plays, painting, graphic design, creative writing, journalism, and other activities that demonstrate you have a creative side.
- **Clubs:** debate, language, chess, multicultural, 4-H, math, National Honor Society, pre-med, junior ROTC, yearbook staff, Audubon Society, and other clubs that you have a keen interest in.
- **Community Service:** Habitat for Humanity, Rotary, key club, Adopt-a-Highway, animal rescue, community outreach, community theater, event planning and organizing, summer camps, church-related activities, and other service for which you did not get paid.
- **Music:** school band, orchestra, chorus, or other music endeavors either at school, at church, or in the community.
- **Student Government:** school council, prom committee, advisory boards, young republicans, young democrats, and any other governance type activity.
- **Sports:** baseball, basketball, football, track, tennis, lacrosse, soccer, swimming, etc.
- **Volunteer Work:** tutoring, hospital work, nursing homework, missionary work, mentoring, homeless shelter, and any other volunteer activity that is not for pay and shows that you care about others and want to make the world a better place.

If you have a job, make sure to include that as part of your activities, but also explain why you may not have had time for other things. And because having a leadership role in extracurricular activities is so important, always emphasize that as well. For example, if you were heading a fund raiser or serving as an officer for a student organization, or took the lead in designing sets for your school's plays, don't be afraid to toot your own horn. Schools want to know that you have passion and talent and are willing to devote your time to excel in something rather than doing activities just because they'll help you get into college.

Improving Test-Taking Skills Now

From the time you enter high school, your grades will depend mainly on tests. Some of these tests will be life changing. The SAT, which determines to a large extent whether or not you're admitted to a select college, exams in your college premed classes that will determine your GPA and ultimately your chances of getting into medical school, and the MCAT, one of the main selection factors in medical school admissions. If you're a good student but a poor test-taker, the odds are against you because, like it or not, your performance in classes will be determined by your ability to do well on tests.

As a college professor for 30 years, I've seen above average students do poorly in class only because they didn't test well. On the other hand, some not so great students did much better than expected because they were particularly good at taking tests. In many cases, just learning the basic techniques that improve test-taking skills can make the difference between success and failure.

It's a shame to see good students who should do much better in class fail just because of poor test-taking skills. The last chapter addresses that, as well as other issues such as study and learning skills, critical thinking, memorization, and overcoming test anxiety. Sometimes becoming an excellent student requires nothing more than a change in attitude and a bit of conditioning. And in many cases, the secret to success is learning how to learn, and learning what it takes to do well on exams.

Accelerated Medical Programs

Accelerated does not mean shortened. While some of these "combined" BA/MD or BS/MD programs are 6 to 7 years long, many are not accelerated at all, and it will still take 8 years to complete. So it's more correct to say that they are combination programs in which students who are serious about medical school are admitted not only to an undergraduate college but to medical school.

This doesn't mean that students who are accepted cannot change their minds and not go to medical school after getting a BS degree. But that's why these programs are so careful in making selections. They don't want to waste time and valuable resources on students who will not continue on to medical school. As an aside, because a premed curriculum is so tough, unless you're a serious student, I would never choose a 6-year program and have to cram all those science courses into two years.

The main criterion for admission into one of these programs is academic excellence. Students are typically in the top 1% of their high school class, take multiple AP courses, and have outstanding SAT scores. Many also participate in scientific research at a local university. Other factors considered are motivation, maturity, character, and strong evidence of extracurricular activities that shows an interest in medicine, such as working at a hospital or shadowing a physician. Because of how competitive these accelerated programs are, applicants must convince committee members that they're serious about a career in medicine.

One of the advantages of accelerated programs is that you don't have to be a science major, as long as you take the prerequisite courses for admission to medical school. This could work to your benefit if you ultimately decide that medicine is not for you. A list of programs can be found by looking at the Association of American Medical Colleges website (www.aamc.org), but it's usually not complete because college curricula change, and programs added. Therefore, it's always best to look at a college's latest catalogue or visit their website to see if it offers an accelerated medical program. A quick review of a college's online catalogue will list the requirements and admissions criteria and help guide you through the application process.

Choosing the Right College

Most medical school admissions committee members will agree that one of the most important factors in the selection process is the undergraduate school you've attended. As a high school student whose goal is getting into medical school, your priority should be to get admitted to the best college you possibly can. That doesn't mean you have to go to a private or an ivy league school. Many public colleges and universities are outstanding and have good records of students getting into medical school. But regardless of whether they are public or private, the most selective colleges will give you the greatest advantage.

Medical school admissions officers are sometimes notorious for rejecting applicants from small, non-competitive schools in favor of those who've graduated from distinguished schools having records of success in placing medical school applicants. This is especially true of medical schools associated with undergraduate institutions that serve almost like feeder programs. One of the main reasons for this is that select colleges with rigorous curricula tend to weed out students who probably wouldn't make it in medical school. Many small colleges may not even have premed advisors, much less entire committees guiding students throughout their first few years of college. Therefore, your number one goal needs to be admission into a select college with a good record of success in placing medical school applicants.

Because the college you attend will be a big factor in your success, find out as much as you can about your college choices. Visit colleges, especially the department that handles the premedical curriculum (usually biology), and insist on answers to these questions:

1. What percent of students who've applied to medical school from your college have gained admission? Find out the actual number of applicants and the number of successful entrants. If a hundred students have applied over the past five years, and only two have been admitted, that's a red flag.
2. What were the academic characteristics (GPA and MCAT scores) of students who've been accepted or rejected by medical schools from your college? Low MCAT scores, for example, may indicate that the academics are not rigorous enough.
3. What kind of premedical program and premedical advising does your college offer?

The reasons for insisting on this information are threefold. Firstly, you need to know a college's track record because that's a good indication of how medical schools view the undergraduate program. Naturally, colleges with rigorous premed programs and proven track records of placing students will always have an advantage. Secondly, the academic credentials of students who do or do not get admitted can give you an idea of a college's reputation. If students with average GPAs are successful in gaining admission to medical school, it's a sure bet that the premed program is difficult, and the level of competitiveness is higher than at other schools. On the other hand, if many students having high GPAs are rejected, the school may not have the reputation of being competitive enough. And thirdly, a college having an established premedical advisory program can offer you more in terms of preparation and development than one lacking such a program.

Don't be afraid to seek out the premedical advisors and ask them as many questions as you think you need to. If a school insists there are no records or information of this kind, or refuses to make them available, you should think twice about applying there. Either the college has a bad record of medical school admissions or the premedical program is not run well enough to have that sort of data available. In both cases, that should serve as a warning sign. Good schools with good records of placing students will proudly offer you all the information you need.

Questions about College Choices

When deciding on a college and a major, especially when that major is going to lead to medical school, high school students invariably have a lot of questions. Many of those questions were probably answered already, but here are some of the most common ones that admissions officers hear year after year.

Q. Is it better to attend a highly competitive college even though my grades may be lower at graduation?

A. Definitely yes, to a point. It won't matter much what college you attend if you graduate with straight C's. However, medical schools are familiar with college reputations, and would rather have a student with good grades in science courses and a 3.4 GPA from a highly selective college than a student with a 3.8 GPA from a least competitive school. Your goal should be to get admitted to the most competitive program you can.

Q. Are there specific colleges that will give me an edge when applying to medical school?

A. When you look at students admitted to medical schools, you'll notice two things:

1. Students with the best chances of admission graduate from highly selective private and public universities. Students from the least selective colleges fared the worst. In fact, the majority of new medical students come from less than 400 colleges nationwide.
2. Medical schools associated with undergraduate programs have a disproportionate number of students who graduate from those programs. What this tells you is that medical schools give preference to their own. So to improve your chances, why not apply to schools that also have medical schools associated with them?

Q. Should I apply to college as a premed major?

A. No. Unless you're applying to an accelerated program that includes admission to medical school, it's not necessary or advisable. I've been around admissions officers and faculty members long enough to know that the term "premed" is sometimes a negative. It's not that colleges don't want students who'll go on to medical school; it's that they'd rather have good all-around students who may eventually apply to medical school regardless of their major. And since the overwhelming number of students will never end up in medical school, colleges are looking for students who have alternate career choices. Once you're accepted, you can major in anything you like anyway.

Q. What is the most important factor that select colleges look for when considering applicants?

A. According to a survey of more than 500 college admissions directors, excellent high school grades and the courses in which they were earned are the most important determining criteria. Difficult AP courses are a must, as are good SAT scores and a record of extracurricular activities. But when pressed to give the top reason for admission, it comes down to good grades in a rigorous curriculum.

Q. How important are extracurricular activities?

A. Students applying to select universities are all going to have good grades and high SAT scores. And since the better schools receive thousands of applications from outstanding students, extracurricular activities and distinguishing characteristics will set you apart. So make sure that you participate in non-academic activities in which you excel and in which you take on leadership roles. That's how you set yourself apart from the rest of the pack and make your application stand out.

Q. What are interviewers looking for when interviewing an applicant?

A. Different interviewers look for different qualities depending on the kind of freshman class the university is looking for. Some admissions officers are looking to increase diversity while others may simply want the best and the brightest. But in general, there are five basic areas all good colleges focus on when conducting interviews. They are:

Intellectual potential: Be prepared to answer questions about your high school courses, favorite books, news events, or anything else that might show intellectual promise. Several days before the interview, look through newspapers and become familiar with recent events. If an opportunity arises for you to mention something in the news, you'll earn points for being well versed.

Motivation: Make a list of accomplishments before the interview and make sure you can talk about them in a way that will demonstrate your drive to be successful. As you list your accomplishments, awards, achievements, etc., be prepared to explain why these were significant and how they prepared you for college.

Maturity: Maintain a relaxed and confident demeanor throughout the interview. Don't make jokes with the interviewer, but don't be somber either. The best way to attack an interview is to answer questions honestly and seriously, but calmly, always maintaining eye contact with the interviewer. Men should wear a conservative suit while women should wear a dress or suit. Remember, first impressions mean a lot, and they set the mood for the rest of the interview.

Leadership: Good schools that receive thousands of applications from excellent students are looking for those intangible qualities that set individuals apart. Leadership is probably number one on the list. When participating in extracurricular activities, strive for leadership roles. When talking about your activities, make sure you emphasize how well you've carried out your responsibilities and leadership roles and how well these have helped you prepare for college.

Overall Image: This is one of those intangible qualities determined by what the interviewer thinks of you as a person. Image may depend on your personality, ability to respond to questions in an intelligent way, body language, honesty, confidence, poise, and articulateness. It's always a good idea to go through several mock interviews to get some feedback on speech problems, annoying habits, or anything else that might ruin an otherwise smooth interview.

Q. How do I know what a college's reputation is for getting students into medical school?

A. The best way to know is to ask the college how many of their graduates were successful in gaining admission to medical school during the past five years. Some schools have great premed programs and great reputations. If a school won't say or tells you it had one student get into medical school during the past 3 to 5 years, it may not be the school you want to depend on for your undergraduate program. Bottom line: if very few students are getting in medical school, it's a good bet that their academics are just not good enough.

Top U.S. Premed Programs

Because students can major in anything they like, as long as they take the required courses needed for admission to medical school, most colleges don't have designated premed programs. The majority of premed students, however, are biology majors because (1) it's a natural transition from biology to medicine, and (2) a biology curriculum generally includes all the classes necessary for the MCAT and for medical school admissions. Although there's no official ranking for premed programs like there is for colleges in general, a few select schools are known for their premedical programs based on exceptional faculty, undergraduate research opportunities, funding, and reputation for getting students accepted to medical school. The following list, which changes annually, includes colleges and universities that have recently been ranked as the best premed programs in the nation:

Amherst College
Brown University
Case Western Reserve University
Columbia University
Cornell University
Duke University
Emory University
Northwestern University
Rice University
Stanford University
Tulane University
University of Chicago
University of North Carolina – Chapel Hill
University of Pennsylvania

Georgetown University
Harvard University
Johns Hopkins University
Vanderbilt University
Washington University
Yale University

Colleges Supplying the Most Applicants to U.S. Medical Schools

The number of applicants a college supplies to medical schools is often a good indicator of how successful its premed program is. There's no guarantee that an applicant from one of these colleges will be admitted to medical school, but it's a good bet that the program is well established and has a good track record. The following is a list of the top 50 colleges in the nation that supply the most applicants each year to medical schools.

Top 50 Colleges Supplying the Greatest Number of Applicants to U.S. Medical Schools	
Undergraduate Institution Rank	**Total No.**
University of California, Los Angeles, CA	1,195
University of Texas, Austin, TX	993
University of Florida, Gainesville, FL	860
University of Michigan, Ann Arbor, MI	824
University of California, Berkeley, CA	735
University of California, San Diego, CA	646
University of Georgia, Athens, GA	591
Texas A&M University, College Station, TX	579
University of North Carolina, Chapel Hill, NC	541
Ohio State University, Columbus, OH	522
University of Virginia, Charlottesville, VA	511
University of Wisconsin, Madison, WI	510
Johns Hopkins University, Baltimore, MD	506
University of California, Davis, CA	481
University of Washington, Seattle, WA	464
Rutgers University, New Brunswick, NJ	442

University of Texas, Dallas, TX	438
University of South Florida, Tampa, FL	438
University of California, Irvine, CA	430
University of Central Florida, Orlando, FL	422
University of Pittsburgh, Pittsburgh, PA	415
University of Maryland, College Park, MD	412
Arizona State University, Tempe, AZ	405
Cornell University, Ithaca, NY	405
Michigan State University, East Lansing, MI	391
Baylor University, Houston, TX	390
University of Minnesota, Minneapolis, MN	384
Emory University, Atlanta, GA	375
Washington University, St. Louis, MO	372
Brigham Young University, Provo, UT	367
University of Illinois - Urbana-Champaign, Champaign, IL	362
Louisiana State University, Baton Rouge, LA	361
University of Southern California, Los Angeles, CA	352
Florida International University, Miami, FL	336
Boston University, Boston, MA	334
University of Pennsylvania, Philadelphia, PA	321
Florida State University, Tallahassee, FL	320
University of Arizona, Tucson, AZ	316
Duke University, Durham, NC	306
Notre Dame University, Notre Dame, IN	298
Stony Brook University, Stony Brook, NY	297
Vanderbilt University, Nashville, TN	292
Indiana University, Bloomington, IN	286
Penn State University, University Park, PA	284

University of California, Riverside, CA	281
University of Miami, Coral Gables, FL	279
University of Houston, Houston, TX	276
Brown University, Providence, RI	267
New York University, New York, NY	266
University of Kentucky, Lexington, KY	261

High School 4-Year Timetable

A common mistake high school students make is waiting until their junior year before making plans for college. Getting into the college of your choice requires that you begin early, preferably in your freshman year. It's much easier to start off right and stay on track than to start slowly and have to catch up. The following is a 4-year timetable that outlines what you need to be doing or thinking about throughout your four years of high school. Use this as a guide after consulting with your school guidance counselor.

Freshman Year

1. Start off right by developing good study habits and time management skills. Also work on your learning, test-taking, and critical thinking skills. When competing with other students who are just as qualified as you, there's no substitute for good grades when applying to college.
2. Study academic requirements of select colleges and plan your academic schedule to be as rigorous as possible, and that includes as many AP classes as you can handle.
3. Participate in no more than two extracurricular activities. It's to your advantage to be committed to a few activities and strive for leadership roles. Spreading yourself out too thin will make it seem as if you're just trying to pad your application with stuff you did.
4. Begin a file of your school activities, volunteer work, jobs, etc.
5. Meet with any college representatives that visit your high school.

Sophomore Year

1. Sign up for the toughest courses you can take, and study hard to get good grades.
2. Continue with your extracurricular activities but focus on achieving high grades. If you must, choose only one activity, do it well, and show commitment and leadership.
3. Continue looking at college programs and begin deciding on some school choices that seem like a good fit for you and your career goals.
4. Study for and take the PSAT. Look at your results and follow suggestions for improvement.
5. Continue your file of extracurricular activities.

6. Meet with college representatives who visit your high school. If you can, visit a college during your break and talk to admissions counselors.

Junior Year

1. Make a tentative list of your top ten college choices and make sure your academic schedule meets their requirements. Take any additional coursework if necessary.
2. Look at college web sites, visit campuses, and get brochures to have as much information as you can about their programs, scholarships, financial aid packages, etc.
3. Study for and take the PSAT. Look at your results and follow suggestions for improvement.
4. Take an SAT prep course or an ACT prep course.
5. Register for the SAT and the ACT.
6. Continue extracurricular activities, but make sure you're consistent in what you're doing. Schools don't like to see a scattergun approach in which you're constantly doing something different. Admissions officers prefer students who choose to do something long-term because it shows commitment and dedication. If your goal is medical school, for example, then volunteering at a nursing home or hospital year after year looks great.
7. Visit prospective colleges during break and talk to admissions counselors.

Senior Year

1. Write, rewrite, edit, and proofread your college essay.
2. Visit colleges and talk to admissions counselors.
3. Prepare for and take the SAT or ACT. Allow plenty of time to study properly because select schools require high SAT scores.
4. Have your FAFSA financial/tax information available to be submitted by January 1.
5. Get letters of recommendation.
6. Forward SAT scores and/or ACT scores to colleges.
7. Fill out applications from colleges of your choice. When writing an essay, do several drafts and then have someone with good editing and proofreading skills check it over for spelling, grammar, punctuation, sentence structure, etc.
8. Fill out financial aid forms and other application materials such as housing, immunization records, etc.
9. Verify with colleges that your application materials are complete.
10. Schedule college interviews.
11. Make a choice and confirm your acceptance.

Beware of senior slump! There's a long-standing tradition in high school that students will spend the last semester taking easy electives and going to gym instead of continuing to work in harder classes. Bad idea. An increasing number of schools, especially more select universities, are catching on to this little scam, and they're rescinding letters of acceptance after reviewing final transcripts. So don't assume that taking a break from school during your last semester is not going to affect your acceptance to college. It very well might. The best strategy is the simplest: don't slack off and don't be tempted to kick back. It's not worth jeopardizing all your effort and hard work for a few months of downtime. You'll have the summer before going off to college to do that.

Many high school students begin college ill-prepared for college-level courses. Don't be one of those students. By starting now, your road through the early years of college – when most premed students drop out or are weeded out – will be easier and much more rewarding. Precollege preparation will give you an advantage over students who'll be overwhelmed and who have never learned to study properly.

CHAPTER 3

THE PREMEDICAL CURRICULUM

As a first-year college student, you have multiple paths to getting into medical school. Majoring in biology, although the most common path, is only one of them. Each year, many non-science majors get accepted because they do well in their required coursework, participate in extracurricular activities that make them stand out, and sell themselves during the interview. If you want to be a doctor, don't think you have to major in biology or chemistry. While the road to medical school is tough, statistics show that anyone with any major can get accepted and do well.

Types of Students Who Should Not Consider Medical School

Before you even consider premed, you need to be honest with yourself, know your abilities and your personality, and do some soul searching. The time commitment involved in a premedical curriculum is more than it is for most college majors. It's not a decision to be made lightly. For many students, premed is so tough they change their career goals after the first year. Although there are exceptions, you probably are not the type of student who should consider medicine as a career if:

1. **You're not a team player.** Although some physicians such as pathologists work behind the scenes, most do not. They're working together with hospital administrators, nurses, other doctors, and office staff. Medicine is a team effort, and unless you're a good communicator and willing to work as a member of a team, medicine may not be a good fit. Medical schools recognize this and are changing curriculums to be more group oriented.
2. **You hate red tape, bureaucracy, and competition.** In medical school, there are no easy days, and many of your classmates will be highly competitive. The first two years are especially stressful, not only because there's so much to learn but also because you've never had to work that hard before. Once you become a physician, the red tape and bureaucracy continues. So, if you're not the type of person who can handle the daily grind, find another career path.
3. **You're not a lifelong learner.** Physicians are students for life. And because medical advances are happening so fast, you'll be left behind and feel incompetent if you don't

keep up with the latest medical therapies and trends. The amount of information is incredible, so unless you look forward to learning for the rest of your life, medicine is the wrong career choice.

4. **You're not willing to put your life on hold until you finish school.** Ask any doctor, and he or she will tell you that medical school is a big sacrifice. You'll have to put lots of things, including family, on hold while you study, cram, and learn.
5. **You're not interested in learning how and why things work.** If you think memorizing facts in college was a big deal, multiply that a thousand times and that's what you'll be doing in medical school. But even though you'll have to memorize countless facts, you'll also have to understand how and why things work. So, for example, if you're not interested in how diseases start, what their mechanisms are, and why therapies work to treat or cure those diseases, then you probably don't have the drive or natural curiosity it takes to be a doctor.
6. **You don't have a love for learning in general.** Some students learn because they must pass exams and get through their courses. Others learn because they love to learn. These are the students who do well in medical school and become good doctors. It goes back to being a lifelong learner. Unless you have a passion to learn and keep learning, you'll not be successful in medicine.
7. **You don't have a strong desire to help others.** For the most part, people become interested in medicine because they have a genuine desire to help others. If your only reason for going to medical school is to have a career in which you make a lot of money, soon you're going to be miserable. The most successful people are the ones who love what they do and, as a result, become great at their jobs.

Beginning Your Premed Strategy

Ideally, premedical planning begins during high school, since getting into the right college is often a steppingstone to successful medical school admissions. Realistically, though, many students are late bloomers, taking general education classes the first year until their interests are channeled in a certain direction. If you're one of those late bloomers, don't worry; the days when medical schools preferred only science majors are long gone. Some medical schools like to have a diverse class, and they recruit good non-science majors into their programs.

One of the major changes in students admitted to medical school is their undergraduate major. The total number of applicants majoring in science has remained steady, but the percentage of non-science majors being admitted has increased. The emphasis on non-science is reflected in the new MCAT, which includes a section called Psychological, Social, and Biological Foundations of Behavior. According to the AAMC, the addition of this section determines an applicant's knowledge of socio-cultural and behavioral aspects of health and health outcomes. And it's one of the reasons some medical schools require applicants to have courses in psychology and/or sociology.

A good strategy is to make sure you have the prerequisites all medical schools require, as well as courses other schools require in addition to those. After all, you're not going to apply to just one or two schools, so make sure that you cover your bases broadly. Take psychology or sociology as electives, for example, because a growing number of medical schools are requiring those as prerequisites. The best way to get an idea of differing requirements is to look at the medical school's web site.

Today's medical schools are looking for well-rounded students who happen to be great in science. After all, you can be the most empathetic and compassionate person in the world, but if you don't have the capacity to learn and understand scientific facts, you're not going to make it through the first year of medical school. They also look for students who, regardless of their major, can show their passion for medicine by having participated in some sort of medically related activity at a hospital, clinic, or doctor's office. Your strategy, then, needs to include not only a strong foundation in the sciences but a resume of activities that prove to admissions officers that you have what it takes to succeed in medical school.

Choosing a Major

Even though most medical school applicants are biology majors, medical schools don't care whether you're a science major or not. In fact, acceptance rates for other majors are just as high, as long as MCAT scores and grades in required science classes are good. For the 2024 class, the highest acceptance rates by major were humanities, physical sciences, and math and statistics, with half of all humanities majors being accepted to at least one medical school. Medical schools realize that a student needs to have an alternate career, just in case. So as long as you complete all the required coursework needed for admission, you should major in anything you like and would enjoy doing in the event you can't get into medical school.

If you do major in something other than science, you can use this to your advantage by showing admissions committees you're mature enough to consider other career options, but are still sincere enough about medical school to complete all the necessary science coursework. Since most medical school applicants are biology and chemistry majors, you may stand out from the pack, as long as you don't neglect the science coursework. You can get straight A's in your major, but if you don't do well in science classes, you're not going to be a good candidate. On the other hand, if you're a History or an English major who gets A's and B's in physics and organic chemistry, you will absolutely impress a medical school admissions committee.

A study that looked at four types of college major clearly showed there were no significant differences in scores on the MCAT. One of the more interesting results in the study was that social science and humanities majors took as little as 40 percent of their credits in science courses compared to 56 percent taken by physical science majors, yet both groups had similar academic performances. In other words, you don't have to give up courses you'd like to take just because you think that taking some extra science classes will help you. They really don't.

A more important, but not surprising fact, was that on the empathy test (designed to measure interpersonal aspects of the doctor-patient relationship), physical science majors scored the lowest while social science majors scored the highest. Considering this, more attention is being given to attitudes and personality traits because a student's major may reveal more about his or her abilities as a future doctor than previously believed. After all, once the details of organic chemistry formulas and physics equations are forgotten, attitudes, sensitivity to interpersonal issues, knowledge of medicine in general, and the ability to develop good doctor-patient relationships are really the critical factors in health care.

So now that you know a science major is not a prerequisite for admission to medical school, you need to understand that there are certain courses all medical schools require and some that most schools require in addition. There are also some courses that medical schools look favorably on even though they're not part of the admissions criteria. Medical school faculty members have told me that certain classes can enhance a student's overall credentials because they demonstrate the student's real interest in science and medicine. The following are examples of premedical curricula at select universities.

Sample Premedical Curriculum for Biology Majors

Freshman Year	English Composition I & II, 6 credit hours
	General Biology I & II w/lab, 8 credit hours
	General Chemistry I & II w/lab, 8 credit hours
	Calculus I, 4 credit hours
	Psychology, 3 credit hours
	Elective, 3 credit hours
Sophomore Year	Organic Chemistry I & II, 8 credit hours
	General Physics I & II, 8 credit hours
	General Microbiology, 4 credit hours
	Statistics, 4 credit hours
	Electives, 6 credit hours
Junior Year	Human Anatomy and Physiology I & II, 8 credit hours
	Molecular Biology, 4 credit hours
	Genetics, 4 credit hours
	Evolutionary Biology, 4 credit hours
	Electives, 9 credit hours
Senior Year	Ecology, 4 credit hours
	Biology electives, 6 credit hours
	Foreign Language, 6 credit hours
	Electives, 9 credit hours

Sample Premedical Curriculum for Non-Science Majors

Freshman Year	Principles of Biology I & II w/lab, 8 credit hours
	General Chemistry I & II w/lab, 8 credit hours
	College Algebra and Pre-calculus, 6 credit hours
	English Composition, 3 credit hours
	History of the Modern World, 3 credit hours
	Introduction to Philosophy, 3 credit hours
	Elective, 3 credit hours
Sophomore Year	Organic Chemistry I & II w/lab, 8 credit hours
	Molecular Biology I & II, 8 credit hours
	Calculus, 4 credits
	Ethics, 3 credits
	History, 3 credits
	English Literature, 3 credits
	Electives, 6 credits
Junior Year	Physics I & II w/lab, 8 credits
	English Literature, 3 credits
	Course in major, 3 credits
	Foreign language I & II, 6 credits
	Social/Behavioral Science, 6 credits
	Philosophy, 3 credits
Senior Year	Course in major, 6 credits
	Fine arts elective, 3 credits
	Upper level biology course, 4 credits
	Foreign language III, 3 credits
	Fine arts and humanities electives, 6 credits
	Free electives, 9 credit hours

These are only two examples of premedical curricula offered at colleges across the nation. Even within departments, curricula may be different depending on whether a student chooses to complete a B.S. or a B.A. degree. The important thing is that you take all the required courses for admission to medical school, as well as courses that will enhance your chances of success. As you can see in both samples, you'll have to take a year of biology and physics and two years of chemistry as your core science classes.

When considering undergraduate schools, choose colleges that have strong premed programs but that also consider a student's desire to major in something other than biology. The best way to do that is to visit the school and talk to advisors in the premed program. One final note: some medical schools take note of the sequence and timing of courses taken in a premed program and take a skeptical view of colleges that delay important courses such as organic chemistry until the junior year. So regardless of which undergraduate school you attend, it's always best to take the required courses during the first two years. Besides, taking all your prerequisite courses before sitting for the MCAT will only help you.

Myths versus Realities of Majoring in Science

Most students make certain assumptions about undergraduate majors and medical school admissions that are simply not true. Ask any guidance counselor and he or she will tell you that your choice of major is not going to affect your chances of getting into medical school. What *will* affect your chances are GPA, MCAT scores, extracurricular activities, and letters of recommendation. Here are a few myths you need to dispel right from the outset:

Myth: majoring in biology will give me an advantage when I apply to medical school.

Reality: medical schools admit students from virtually every major. In fact, today's medical schools are looking for a diverse student body with a variety of undergraduate experiences. Admissions committee members are also aware that even qualified candidates may not be accepted and, therefore, students need to have a plan B in case they don't get in. The reality is that you'll do much better in college if you love what you're studying, no matter what major it is.

Myth: graduating with a double major will look good on my application.

Reality: this is not necessarily true, especially if your grades are not that good. It doesn't matter if you double major in biology and chemistry if you graduate with a 2.75 GPA. An English major with a 3.75 GPA, which includes all the medical school prerequisites, is considered head and shoulders above a double major with a 3.0 GPA.

Myth: because it took me 5 years to complete my degree, I'm at a disadvantage.

Reality: there's no rule that says you must apply to medical school after your junior year in order to get in that following year. Sometimes that extra year will help you prepare better for the MCAT, which is critically important for admissions. Medical schools don't see this as a negative, and may actually view you as more mature and conscientious, especially if you've been working while going to school or had some extraordinary issues that kept you from graduating in four years.

Myth: taking difficult science courses in college will get me into medical school.

Reality: if you can take several difficult science classes a semester and do well, your chances are great. However, if taking a lot of hard classes gets you straight C's, you're out of luck, no matter how many classes you take. Bottom line: grades count, not the number of classes you take.

Myth: if I take one science course per semester or take a tough class like organic chemistry in the summer, I can focus on getting good grades and becoming more competitive.

Reality: admissions committees will see you as a weak applicant who has not taken a rigorous or challenging number of courses each semester. Their thinking will be that if you lighten your load just so you'll get better grades, how are you going to handle medical school, which is much more challenging than anything you'll experience in college.

Required Courses for Admission

Because medical schools determine their own entrance requirements, including prerequisite coursework, you must check the requirements and the rules for acceptable courses for every school to which you plan to apply. In addition, almost every school requires the MCAT; and the required courses you'll have to take for admission are necessary for you to do well on the entrance exam. The required courses for most medical schools are:

- 1 year of Biology with lab
- 1 year of Inorganic Chemistry with lab
- 1 year of Organic Chemistry with lab
- 1 year of Physics with lab
- 1 year of English

Some schools also require calculus, statistics, or other college level math; and many require biochemistry, psychology, and/or sociology. Some other recommended courses medical schools like to see on a student's transcript are Genetics, Anatomy & Physiology, Molecular Biology, and Computer Science. Check the school catalogue for specific requirements. Furthermore, because the new MCAT includes a good deal of biochemistry and a section on Psychological, Social, and Biological Foundations of Behavior, your undergraduate curriculum should include courses in those as well.

Traditionally, organic chemistry has been the "weed out" course that keeps students out of medical school. One faculty member told me that getting a C in organic chemistry can really hurt a student's chances. Many hopeful premeds that do well in biology and math drop organic chemistry and change majors within a month of registering for it, so it's important to start strong and not fall behind.

Why Organic Chemistry is the Weed-Out Course for Premeds

Ask any premed student and most will tell you that organic chemistry, especially organic chemistry II, is the toughest course they've taken in college. At some schools, professors take pride in making this a weed-out course for potential medical students; and I've personally known good students who've given up on medicine because of organic chemistry.

There are a few reasons for this. At one large university, where a thousand freshmen wanted to go into medicine, a professor actually said that he needed to weed out as many of the weak students as possible to make the advising and the application process more manageable. What school, according to the professor, wants to have hundreds of weak applicants who have no chance of getting into medical school? Another reason is that organic chemistry requires more study time than just about any other course, and naturally the weak students will drop out. If a student can't spend 10 or more hours a week studying for a single course, there's no way he or she is going to get through medical school.

The reason admissions committees look closely at organic chemistry grades is because organic chemistry requires not only memorization (although some claim it does not) and lots of study time, but problem-solving skills. Even though you won't have to know much organic chemistry as a physician, the fact that you're able to do well in the course says a lot about 1) your study habits, 2) your motivation, drive, and determination, and 3) your problem solving skills.

An A or B in organic chemistry tells the admissions committee members that you have what it takes to get through a tough medical school curriculum. One of the reasons students do poorly in organic chemistry is that they have a preconceived notion that it's the toughest course they'll ever take. That may be true for some, but many students do very well in organic chemistry and find it fun and challenging. It doesn't have to be the hell-on-earth class everyone dreads and that many students fail. It could actually be the course that makes you a much better applicant and helps you do well on the MCAT. The following are six ways to make organic chemistry easier and keep it from being the weed-out course that keeps you out of medical school:

- **Don't believe the hype.** Many students go into organic chemistry scared out of their wits simply because they've been told that it's the toughest course they'll ever encounter. Some professors also scare students into believing this. Although it is a tough course, it doesn't have to be any more difficult than other science classes, if you apply yourself and study hard. The material to be mastered in organic chemistry doesn't change, only the way professors teach it. So go into the class expecting to spend a lot of time studying and reviewing, and then study.
- **Study hard and study every day.** The only way to get an A in organic chemistry is to spend at least 10 hours a week studying. If you're not used to spending that much time on a single course, get used to it because it's quite easy to fall behind and get lulled into a false sense of security. Organic chemistry requires that you study and review every single day so that the material becomes familiar and less intimidating.
- **Understand, don't memorize.** One of the biggest mistakes students make when learning organic chemistry is trying to memorize everything. Naturally, there will be memorization involved, but more important is your ability to really understand what's going on so that you can solve problems you've never seen before. Each concept in organic chemistry builds upon previous principles, so get in the habit of reviewing summaries and notes from previous material as new material is introduced.
- **Draw out mechanisms.** Even if you don't have to draw out mechanisms to get an

answer, do so anyway. By drawing mechanisms, you'll get a better understanding of the chemistry involved and you'll become more intuitive. One of the best books I've seen for helping students visualize organic molecules is *Pushing Electrons* by Daniel Weeks.

- **Work as many problems as possible.** It's not enough to read and understand the material. You must work lots of problems in order to apply the concepts you learn. Always study with a pencil and paper, and never resort to the answer page until you have seriously attempted to solve the problem. When you get an answer wrong, understand why. It's not enough to read through problems and look at the answers. You must do the problems.
- **Work in groups.** Organic chemistry is one of those courses where it helps to study in groups. Ask each other questions, solve problems together, and teach one another. If you can explain a concept to someone else, then you know that you understand it.
- **Don't wait to get help.** Falling behind is one the biggest reasons for failure, so as soon as you encounter problems, go see the instructor or tutor for help. Don't underestimate the value of extra help sessions. If they're offered, go to them, ask questions, and review what you've learned. It's hard to catch up in organic chemistry once you've fallen behind, so the best way to do well is to try to get ahead of the class and look for help at the first sign of trouble.

The way in which you learn and practice organic chemistry will be beneficial to the way you'll learn material in medical school. Courses such as biochemistry, pharmacology (which has a lot of organic compounds), microbiology, and pathology all involve concepts that build on each other, much like in organic chemistry. Perhaps that's why admissions committees believe that doing well in organic prepares you for the way you'll have to think and approach classes in medical school.

Valuable Non-Science Courses

According to Dr. Pellegrino, writing in the Journal of the American Medical Association, "The central act of medicine – making a clinical decision – is only part scientific. To make a right and good decision for a particular patient requires thinking more properly derived from the liberal arts and humanities." And the conclusion of a Rockefeller Foundation-sponsored conference on liberal arts and premedical education was that overemphasizing technical expertise has harmful effects on premed and medical education. Today's medical schools are embracing those findings and implementing a more broadly based undergraduate curriculum. So, in addition to the required science and math courses, there are some humanities, social science, and behavioral courses that look favorably on your transcript. They are: Sociology, Psychology, Philosophy and Ethics, Anthropology, and Behavioral Sciences.

Don't neglect these courses just because you think that you'll never use them in the medical profession. The well-rounded student all medical schools are looking for will certainly be conversant with many of these subjects. They may even come up during your medical school interview or on the MCAT. So it's to your advantage to introduce yourself to the humanities, if for no other reason than to become a better physician. Nothing destroys a doctor-patient relationship faster than a doctor's inability to relate to his or her patient. Medical schools recognize the importance of personal attributes and look for applicants they feel will be both physician and humanitarian.

Although science is essential to medicine, studies in the social sciences and humanities are equally important for a thorough understanding of contemporary society. Physicians must draw upon history, economics, philosophy, and the culture of people to appreciate the many dimensions of human behavior and human problems. They cannot be narrow-minded individuals and be effective in treating patients. Premedical education must prepare you to understand both the scientific and the personal side of human suffering, and to do this you need to blend the study of science with the study of humanities.

The concept of being both healer and humanitarian is so important that the American Board of Internal Medicine has added a requirement to its certification process. New applicants taking the specialty exam in Internal Medicine must be certified by the director of his/her residency program as demonstrating humanistic qualities. As a premed student, then, it would be to your advantage to take some extra humanities classes throughout your undergraduate years.

Reading Scientific Literature

As a medical student, and then later as a physician, you'll have to read an incredible amount of scientific material. Even as a premed, you'll be expected to read scientific articles in many of your classes. At first, this will seem overwhelming because, like most students, you're probably not used to reading scientific literature or science journal articles. This will have to change if you're going to do well in a premedical curriculum. By learning how to read scientific articles, you'll not only do much better in your undergraduate classes, but you'll also improve your performance on the MCAT and be much better prepared for the reading you'll have to do in medical school.

Reading science articles requires a set of rules and a different mindset about what to look for and how to approach the writing. For example, the worst approach is to read the article word for word from title to literature cited as if you were reading a chapter in a textbook. In most cases, all you want is the barebones information, and not waste your time with extraneous details. Here are the rules to follow whenever you're reading any scientific paper:

1. **Read the title carefully and look for key words.** The title should tell you exactly what the article is about and what you'll expect when you begin reading. It should grab your attention immediately and help clarify what to look for.
2. **Read and understand the abstract completely.** Read this part slowly. The abstract always lets you know **why** the research was done (the objectives), **why** it is important, and **what** was found. Basically it's a 200-word summary of the research. In many cases, unless you need the actual details of the research, just reading the

abstract may be enough. If it's not, the next step is to check out the graphs, figures, illustrations, and tables, which should explain what you just read.

3. **Examine the figures and tables.** Before you look at the artwork, it may be necessary to examine the methods and materials, especially if you're interested in the techniques used to conduct the research. If not, skim the methods sections and go on. As you look at the graphs, figures, and tables, study them and understand how they relate to what you read in the abstract.
4. **Go back and read the introduction.** The introduction explains **who** did the research, **when** it was done, **why** it was important, and **what** to expect in the body of the paper. Most importantly, it clearly states why the research was done and why you should care. It also helps you focus on the results to come.
5. **Check the results section.** This section presents the data, period. Look for consistency between the results presented and the figures or tables. You should be able to go back and forth smoothly from reading to looking at figures.
6. **Read the discussion.** Once you've seen the results, the discussion explains how the results compare with the objectives and the hypothesis. This is the most important section because it explains why the researchers got the results they did.
7. **Read the entire article.** Go back and read the article in its entirety. By now, you should have a clear idea of what the article is about. If it's an article that was assigned in class, you may want to read it several times to make sure you understand what it says. Jotting down notes in the margins, circling words, and underlining key phrases will help.
8. **Reread the abstract.** Abstracts are dense and sometimes difficult to read the first time through. To get a firm grasp of exactly what the entire article is about, reread the abstract one more time. After going through the sections of the article several times, this final pass should be much easier and will clear up any questions you may have had.
9. **Look at the citation index.** Lastly, if you find something interesting in an article, you can look up cited references to add to your knowledge base.

Reading a journal article is not like reading a novel. The information is complex and written in jargon you may not fully understand. There's nothing wrong with reading an article several times. I'm always amazed at what I discover the second or even third time I go through a paper. Some articles will be easier to read than others. If the paper is exceptionally long, you may be able to skip over the methods and materials section unless that's important to you. With some papers, you might be able to get the main idea by simply reading the abstract and discussion and looking at the figures.

Spending some time reading a variety of articles – from both scientific journals and popular magazines – will make reading them seem easy. Most journals require subscriptions, but a few will allow you to read full articles after they've been in press for 3 months to a year. Get in the habit of reading a few articles a week and you'll be surprised at how good you become at skimming over the parts you don't feel are important and focusing in on those that are. Here are some great websites to visit if you want to enhance your reading skills:

Popular Science Magazines	**Scientific Journals and Databases**
www.livescience.com	www.core.com
www.nature.com	www.doaj.com
www.newscientist.com	www.epic.ed.gov
www.sciencedaily.com	www.plos.org
www.sciencedirect.com	www.scienceopen.com
www.sciencemag.org	www.ssrn.com

Team-Based Learning and Tutoring

Today's medical schools are taking a team approach to medical education because the highest quality clinical care is delivered not by single doctors but by teams where there's communication, cooperation, and interaction. So rather than learning as individuals, medical students are spending less time in lecture halls and more time learning as groups that interact and work together on projects using team-based learning. As more medical schools implement this system, students who aren't willing to work together or who insist on going it alone will not be successful. Because team-based learning is a growing trend in medical education, you'll be at an advantage if you get used to the process during college.

One of the benefits of working with your peers during college is that you'll demonstrate to potential medical schools that you're a team player and that you'll be a good fit for their program. Medical schools don't want loners who'll spend hours by themselves in a library with no interaction with other students. They expect their students to be social and to work together for the benefit of the group. In fact, entire new medical school facilities are being built with this concept in mind.

The old standard in education was to be competitive, follow the rules, memorize, look for cues to get answers, and be individually responsible. The new standard is to be cooperative, explore, use critical thinking skills, and interact with other students. A good place to start, if you want to build your team learning skills, is to get involved with other students in class projects, and by tutoring. It's said that we learn only 50 percent of what we see and hear but 70 percent of what we discuss and 90 percent of what we teach to others. Tutoring other students is not only a great way to get involved in class but it's the best way to learn just about anything.

Overall Academic Characteristics

If there's a single academic characteristic medical schools are looking for in applicants, besides excellent grades in the general science requirements, it's a broad educational base. Humanities (arts, philosophy, and literature) are important in understanding people, and in developing a more cultured and diverse background. Communication skills – both oral and written – are without question one of the most important criteria in the selection process because they're critical in a physician's ability to interrelate with others. Behavioral sciences are vital in developing a physician's awareness of human personality and the needs of the community, as well as society.

In essence, your undergraduate curriculum must not only show that you're interested in science but that you seek to expand your cultural base and broaden your horizons. Intellect is only part of being a physician. Society places a physician in high regard and, therefore, medical schools accept applicants they feel will represent their programs and their profession in the highest tradition. According to the president of a major university, medicine is so diverse that it can benefit from all kinds of backgrounds and interests.

To give you an idea of how important this philosophy is becoming for medical schools in the future, the Association of American Medical Colleges has made five recommendations for medical school admissions policies. They are:

1. All college and university students should be required to study broadly the natural and social sciences and the humanities.
2. Medical school faculties should require only essential courses and should stop recommending additional courses beyond these.
3. College faculties should make scholarly endeavor and the development of effective communication skills integral features of undergraduate curricula.
4. Medical schools should use admissions criteria that appraise independent learning, analytical and critical thinking skills, and the development of attitudes and values essential for those in a caring profession who are to contribute to the welfare of society.
5. Communication between college and medical school faculty concerning admissions criteria should be improved.

These premedical guidelines are being emphasized because, to understand and have sympathy for those who seek help, the medical association feels that a physician must be deeply attentive to varieties of human behavior, experiences, and personalities. Being a non-physician, therefore, is just as important at times as being a physician. Students selected as future doctors must exhibit all these traits.

A good way to gauge the success of premedical programs is to find out how practicing physicians feel about their college educations. When a recent survey was done in which participating physicians were asked how they felt about the emphasis placed on premedical science and non-science courses, an overwhelming 72 percent said that more emphasis should have been placed on non-science courses in college, especially humanities like English, literature, and philosophy. One physician thought that the chemistry and physics were not all that important in his studies, another said that the humanities were the best preparation for the practice of medicine, and others urged students to do intensive study in literature and the arts. This survey of practicing doctors clearly showed that something was lacking in premedical education.

Once a student enters medical school, the opportunities for a broad liberal education dwindle. After the rigors of medical training and residency, many physicians find that something is lacking in their educational background. By then, the demands of a doctor's life don't leave much room for much else. What these physicians were saying is that, although science is essential in the medical school admissions process, and in medical school education, you need to look ahead and prepare yourself for life beyond medical school. And according to many of these doctor's, humanities are one of the most important ways to do that.

Getting a Head Start on Coursework

Every medical school has specific requirements for admission, but a few medical schools require additional courses. More than 50 require one or more semesters of calculus and/or statistics, more than 30 require biochemistry, which is included on the new MCAT, some require more than a year of biology, and many require psychology or sociology. The current edition of the AAMC's Medical School Admission Requirements gives the latest information on each school's specific criteria. Don't wait until you're well into your premedical curriculum to get details about the medical school you're interested in. By checking requirements, you can begin taking required courses early and give yourself the flexibility to take additional classes to build your credentials.

One of the mistakes students make is not following an organized schedule of courses. They may want to put off organic chemistry or physics, for example, so they can focus on general education requirements and getting their GPA's up. That's a big mistake. Typically, premed programs start you off with the required courses in the very first semester of your freshman year for three important reasons:

1. Typically, you take the MCAT in the spring of your junior year. By taking all the coursework that's covered on the exam, you'll have enough time to study and review and be much better prepared. Statistics show that juniors perform best on the MCAT because the material is still fresh and familiar to them.
2. Any additional coursework you take will not only build your credentials but may help you perform better on the MCAT. Advanced courses naturally build on introductory courses and force you to review concepts you may have forgotten or didn't quite understand the first time.
3. Medical school curricula are rigorous. It would be to your advantage to take some advanced courses in biology such as molecular biology or biochemistry to prepare yourself for the avalanche of information you'll be required to know as a first-year medical student. I've spoken to medical students who've taken biochemistry, genetics, and advanced physiology before entering medical school, and they all told me that it was extremely helpful to have had them.

Having been an advisor for many years, believe me when I tell you that one of the biggest problems I've seen is students falling behind because they procrastinate or rearrange schedules. Colleges know what they're doing when they put together curricula. Certain courses are prerequisites to others, and you need to realize from day one that following a specific schedule will not only guarantee that you stay on track but that you're well prepared for the MCAT. Whether you think you need to or not, getting a head start on your coursework and doing everything you need to do to get into medical school means paying regular visits to your premed advisor.

Why GPA is Important

Medical schools are incredibly competitive, and most applicants have high GPAs. Needless to say, you must have a strong GPA to be considered because GPA is probably the single most important factor in successful admissions. Most premed students graduate with at least a 3.5 GPA, and unless your MCAT scores are high, a low GPA is going to raise some red flags. This is especially true if you attend a school with a reputation for grade inflation. For example, if everyone at a certain school graduates with a minimum GPA of 3.2, your 3.4 GPA is barely above the minimum and is not going to look particularly good.

GPA is important for three reasons. One, grades are really the only way to quantify academic performance against others in your class. If you make C's in all your science classes, it's an indication that you probably won't do well on more difficult exams throughout medical school. Two, four-year graduation and dropout rates are much higher for students with GPAs below 3.0, whereas medical school graduation rates are above 90 percent for students with 3.0 to 4.0 GPAs. And three, your GPA is often seen as a reflection of your work ethic. When someone looks at a student's low GPA, they immediately think that he or she just didn't work hard enough. I've had many bright students who graduated with 2.8 GPAs and many average but hard-working students who graduated with 3.5 GPAs and ended up in medical school.

If you look at the grades of students who've been successful in getting into medical school, less than 5 percent had C averages, and those few had exceptional MCAT scores. High grades, on the other hand, can have a positive effect on lower MCAT scores. If your MCAT scores are not that great, but your GPA is high, it could mean the difference between an interview or not.

Despite the emphasis on grades, premedical GPAs are not always the number one criterion for admissions. For instance, three students I helped get admitted to medical school all had GPAs of around 3.0, and they're all practicing physicians now. Obviously, other factors came into play that helped overcome low grades. These students all had terrific extracurricular activities, and they did well on their MCAT. These are the exceptions. The fact is that to be competitive and to improve your chances of admission, you need to maintain a high GPA.

There's one other factor about grades I feel is important. Admissions committees take other things into consideration when selecting students who don't have very high GPAs. A student may have experienced extraordinary circumstances that prevented him or her from doing as well in school (having to work 40 hours a week to support a family, for example). In the end, though, the rule of thumb is that too many C's hurt, B's don't hurt but can help, and A's definitely increase your odds.

How Anyone Can Be a Genius

Because they must take such difficult courses, premed students work harder and study more than most other students. In addition, they must take the MCAT, which means they also must spend at least three months preparing for that. With so much time devoted to study and learning, and with so much riding on their grades, students in a premed curriculum must develop expert study skills and condition themselves to be continual learners.

Dr. Diola Bagayoku, a Professor of Physics at Southern University, has shown mathematically that, just like athletes increase their performance through training and practice, students can do the same thing with their study. According to Dr. Bagayoku, "Genius is mostly the result of sustained, competitive practice." His studies have shown that academic proficiency is related to adequate practice. In other words, practice makes perfect in everything you do, including learning.

The Power Law of Human Performance states that the time it takes you to perform a task decreases as the number of times you practice that task increases. In other words, if you want to become a genius, you need to train like an Olympic athlete. You must have high expectations and give one hundred percent effort to your study. Practice does make perfect, both in sports and in the classroom. So regardless of race, sex, or age, every student can achieve academic excellence.

Over the years, I've seen average premed students who worked hard and learned how to study outperform even the most talented students because they were willing to put in the effort. If you're serious about medical school, and all that it entails, why would you not train yourself to be the best you could be? Hard work, motivation, and extra effort can more than make up for less talent and intelligence. In fact, according to Dr. Bagayoku, working harder than you've ever worked before might just make you a genius.

Avoiding Premed Syndrome

Medical schools are increasingly on the lookout for students afflicted with something called "premed syndrome." It begins early in a student's undergraduate years and gets progressively worse by the third year of college. Not all students fall victim, but as a faculty member who had to interact with lots of premed students I've seen my share firsthand. The symptoms include: being an ultra-competitive workaholic who argues over every point on an exam, will do whatever it takes to get better grades, will volunteer for activities he or she has no time for and then abandons them just to get something on their resume, are perfectionists, and games the system in order to gain an unfair advantage over his or her classmates.

It seems that the drive to get into medical school and the competition for top grades becomes so intense that premed students develop an attitude totally opposite of what's considered important to becoming a doctor. According to many advisors, faculty, and fellow students, premed students can be excessively grade conscious, narrow in interests, narcissistic, less sociable, more aggressive, and more interested in money or prestige. Many premeds become so narrow minded they plan their entire second and third years around the MCAT and the admissions process. They alter study habits, lighten course loads, refuse to take any class that will affect their GPA, withdraw from extracurricular activities, and pass up work opportunities. In essence, they give up a wonderful and crucial part of their education just to do well on one exam.

There's a well-known formula in the medical school admissions game: grades + MCAT scores + extracurricular activities = admission to medical school. Many premed students take easy courses to get A's and overload on science courses, thinking that getting A's in lots of "other classes" and taking one science course after another is their ticket to medical school. Rather than taking classes that will make them better doctors, they take classes only to help them do well on the MCAT. Some medical schools, unfortunately, still look for aggressive and highly competitive students because these are the types of students who are highly motivated and do well under pressure. However, many more schools are looking at these qualities as negative personality traits and, instead, are leaning toward more broad-minded and people-oriented candidates. That's why students who are non-science majors and who get good grades and MCAT scores have high admission rates and do very well in medical school. They also make great physicians.

All too often, students get incomplete advice from counselors who are not familiar with medical school trends and new medical school admissions requirements. This is especially true at colleges that don't have established premed programs. Regardless of what college you attend, pay a visit early on to a premedical school advisor at your school or at the nearest school that has one. Premed advisors are in contact with medical schools in the area and can give you valuable information about specific and differing requirements.

The key is to begin now. I've talked to many college seniors who regret not having started a plan of action sooner. If there's anything I can't emphasize enough it's the importance of not waiting until it's too late. The sooner you get started, the better off you'll be. And don't assume that being a good student is enough. Medical schools don't want excellent students who have nothing to show but the fact that they'd spent four years only studying. Your plan of action needs to include other areas of accomplishment besides academics for you to develop into the well-rounded student medical schools are looking for. By starting a plan of action from the first semester of college, and staying on track, your chances for admission will improve significantly.

CHAPTER 4

THE APPLICATION PROCESS

After a slight decline in previous years, by 2023 a record number of students (55,188) applied to medical school. Those applicants sent out more than 990,000 applications or an average of 18 applications per student. Several new schools are either being built or in the planning stages. That doesn't mean admission to medical school will be getting any easier; it means that the demand is growing, and more qualified students are considering a career in medicine. Because of increased competition, the need to focus on your application is greater than ever.

The medical school application and admissions process has changed over the years, partly because of increases in the number of medical school applicants, but also because medical education is evolving, and the applicant pool must evolve with it. The selection process in 2024-25 and beyond will see changes due to a revised MCAT, new trends in how medicine is taught, and a focus on selecting students who'll succeed in a dynamic healthcare climate. But despite the changes, every medical school has maintained its own strategy for identifying and selecting what they hope is their ideal medical student. The guidelines in this chapter are followed by most admissions committees, and they should help you understand and prepare for the application process.

Where and When to Begin

The best way to begin is by looking at the most recent issue of the Medical School Admission Requirements, published by the AAMC, or by going to their web site at www.aamc.org. The website doesn't have a great deal of information about specific medical school programs (you must visit the school's website for that), but it's an excellent source of information about the application process. For anyone serious about medical school, the AAMC's site and book are indispensable.

The application process is not all that complicated; it's just that each step involves rules and a timetable that must be followed if you're going to stay on course and complete all the requirements. It's not a sprint, as they say, but a 4-year marathon that requires you to pay attention to course work, due dates, and other activities necessary to build your credentials and complete your application. And that means you need to begin planning the very first semester you start college. The following is a typical 4-year timeline that will ensure progress every step of the way:

Freshman Year

- Meet with a premedical advisor and make sure you understand the premedical curriculum and general medical school admissions requirements.
- Meet with your academic advisor about selecting a sequence of classes.
- Take required prerequisite courses such as biology, inorganic chemistry, and mathematics.
- Seek research opportunities on campus.
- Develop relationships with faculty members who might write future letters of recommendation.
- Begin extracurricular activities and community service.
- Join a premed club or student leadership organization.
- Apply to summer enrichment programs or to summer research programs

Summer

- Participate in summer research or enrichment programs.
- Do volunteer work in a health-related field.

Sophomore Year

- Meet regularly with your premedical advisor.
- Take required prerequisite courses such as organic chemistry and physics, as well as additional courses required by many medical schools. Check individual school catalogues for specific requirements.
- Continue to participate in extracurricular activities as well as community service.
- Engage in a health profession experience such as volunteering at a hospital or clinic or shadowing a physician.
- Apply for a summer research program or internship.

Summer

- Become familiar with the American Medical College Application Service (AMCAS) application process.
- Participate in summer research or enrichment programs.
- Do volunteer work in a health-related field.

Junior Year

- Meet regularly with your premedical advisor to discuss remaining coursework and to go over the timeline and important dates for application.

Fall Semester

- Take additional science and non-science classes as required by

select medical schools.
- Gather information about potential medical schools.
- Decide which faculty members you'll ask for letters of recommendation.
- Prepare for the MCAT. Visit www.aamc.org/mcat to find test dates and locations.
- Register for the Spring MCAT.
- Continue to engage in extracurricular activities and volunteer work in a clinical setting.

Junior Year
- Meet regularly with your premedical advisor.
- Take the MCAT.

Spring Semester
- Begin writing the personal statement.
- Request letters of evaluation.
- Finalize your list of medical schools, which should include both state schools and more select national schools.
- Request a copy of your transcripts required by most medical schools.
- Begin working on the AMCAS application. Make sure you know the deadline dates for every school on your list.
- Continue to engage in extracurricular activities and volunteer work.

Summer
- Complete the AMCAS application.
- If needed, retake the MCAT.
- Continue with extracurricular and volunteer work.

Senior Year
- Meet regularly with your premedical advisor to discuss letters of recommendation and other premedical committee activities.

Fall Semester
- Submit the AMCAS application. Deadlines continue from August through December.
- Complete all degree requirements.
- If medical schools are interested, they'll ask that you submit secondary applications with additional information and essays. Prepare these carefully.
- Prepare for the medical school interviews, which begin as early as August and continue through the spring.
- Continue with extracurricular and volunteer work.
- Wait for notification from medical schools and schedule interviews.

- If you're waitlisted, update medical schools with any additional new accomplishments that may enhance your chances for admission.

Senior Year
- Go on medical school interviews.

Spring Semester
- Make a final decision on which medical school you'll attend.
- Notify medical schools before the deadline that you'll not be attending.
- If not accepted to any medical school, apply again next year.

The general rule is to apply one year before the date that you will be starting medical school. It's important to pay attention to school application dates and deadlines, and to know that medical schools will not review your application unless your MCAT scores are available for them to examine. Premed advisors are especially important during your third year of college because they'll help guide you through the process.

It's also important that you apply as early during the application process as possible because the peak time at most medical school admissions offices is September through December. Once applications begin rolling in, the entire process slows down and there's always that improbable chance that some part of your application will not get to where it's supposed to get. This rarely happens, but I would recommend getting everything in at the beginning. And since most schools don't start processing applications until all the materials are on file, you can rectify any problems with transcripts, letters of recommendation, etc. in plenty of time for proper evaluation.

American Medical College Admissions Service (AMCAS)

AMCAS is a service run by the AAMC in which students use a common online application to apply to U.S. medical schools. It is in no way involved in the selection process. All medical schools except for some schools in Texas, which use the Texas Medical & Dental Schools Application Service (TMDSAS), as well as a few others, participate in AMCAS. Osteopathic schools use a similar application service called the American Association of Colleges of Osteopathic Medicine Application Service or AACOMAS.

To make the application process more streamlined and consistent, AMCAS uses a centralized system that collects all the required materials and information from applicants around the country, verifies it, reviews it line by line, and sends it off to prospective medical schools. Therefore, no matter how many medical schools you apply to, all you must do is submit one online application and one set of letters of recommendation. Because the AMCAS instructions are specific to each application cycle, it's important that you and your premed advisor stay current on the latest version. Everything you'll need to know about AMCAS and the application process, including due dates and the Fee Assistance Program for students in financial need, is available on www.aamc.org/amcas.

AMCAS is not affiliated with any medical school. Its only function is to act as an intermediary between you and whichever medical schools you designate on the application. The concept is especially useful, since you won't have to send individual applications to every school you apply to. Today's online application is much more efficient than it was in the past, but you still need to familiarize yourself with the procedure before you get started.

The AMCAS verification process doesn't begin until all your transcripts are received, and you've completed the entire application. Because staff does a line-by-line review of each section of the application, this can take as long as 6 weeks, especially if it's during the peak season; so it's a good idea to begin planning well in advance and then submit your application as soon as you can. If something is missing or needs to be changed, you'll have plenty of time to address any problems. MCAT scores are automatically forwarded to medical schools, so you don't need to have those before submitting the application. To download the AMCAS instruction manual, go to https://www.aamc.org/students/applying/amcas and click on the instruction manual link.

The Nine-Step Application

The process itself is straightforward since the online site takes you through each section step-by-step. However, you'll have to certify that you've read the AMCAS instruction manual when you submit your application. To register, go on the AMCAS site and create a username and password. If you had already registered for the MCAT or the Fee Assistance Program, you won't have to register again. When you log into your account, the site will guide you through the process. Here's an overview of the nine sections you'll have to complete and suggestions on how to make sure your application is as good as it could be.

Section 1: Identifying Information. This first section asks for your legal name, alternate name, any ID numbers that would help in matching you with the application, birth date, state of birth, sex, and other personal information. Make sure that all this information is complete and accurate before continuing to the next section.

Section 2: Schools Attended. In this section, you'll list your high school, each post-secondary school attended or were enrolled in for at least one course, and any degrees you earned or will be earning. There's a section for students who've been home schooled, who've received a GED, or attended schools outside the U.S. This section also allows you to print transcript request forms to send to all schools from which AMCAS requires transcripts. It's important that you use the official AMCAS transcript request form because AMCAS is not responsible for any transcript they cannot match to your application. It's also important that you inform your school's registrar that the AMCAS transcript request form be attached to the official transcript. Request personal transcript copies for yourself so that you can refer to them when you're completing section 4. For a complete description and information about transcripts, read section 2 of the AMCAS instruction manual.

Section 3: Biographic Information. This section asks for information such as name, address, citizenship, legal residence, primary language, race, dependents, parent's names, military service, and any felonies or misdemeanors. Be careful on this section, and don't be deceptive. If you leave something out, the verification process will usually uncover it.

Section 4: Course Work. As you examine your transcripts, enter all the course work for which you've enrolled at colleges in the U.S., U.S. territories, and Canada. Include courses that you registered for but did not complete, or courses from which you withdrew. Don't omit any coursework! If you do, it will affect and delay your application, which could result in missed deadlines. A complete description of how your coursework should be listed is included in the AMCAS instruction manual.

Section 5: Work and Activities. This section offers students the opportunity to list any work experience, volunteer and extracurricular activities, awards and honors, and publications. A total of 15 experiences are allowed, and they're listed in chronological order. Work experiences and activities are selected from a drop-down list that best describes the type of activity. You'll need to include, among other things, names and addresses of the organizations, dates, and the number of hours you participated.

Because you'll have to provide contact information, keep a list of individuals you worked with so that medical schools can verify you did the activity. One of the most important parts of section 5 is the experience description, where you'll have an opportunity to describe what you've done in about 700 characters. You can identify up to three activities that were most meaningful. Do an excellent job on this part (be clear and concise) because what you've done outside of class could make the difference between getting an interview or not. Spend time rewriting, editing, and proofreading your descriptions.

Section 6: Letters of Evaluation. In this section, you'll list names of individuals who will be writing your letters of evaluation. It's important that you select individuals who can vouch for your work ethic, personal qualities, intellect, and character. Up to ten letters are allowed (not to the same school), which can be individually targeted to different schools. Once the application is processed, letters are automatically submitted to medical schools.

Section 7: Medical Schools. From a drop-down list, you will select, either by the name of the school or the state, the medical schools to which you're applying. Review this part carefully because once you've submitted your application, the names of medical schools cannot be removed or changed. You can, however, add schools to your list if you meet the deadline for application. This section also has a **Show Details** button, which displays information about each of the schools you've designated.

Section 8: Essay. This section requires that you submit a personal essay in which you can distinguish yourself from other applicants. Four important topics to address in your essay are (1) the reason(s) you've chosen medicine as a career, (2) what challenges, hardships, and obstacles you faced to get where you are today, (3) reasons for any gaps in your education or discrepancies in your grades that may be explained by extraneous circumstances, and (4) your primary motivation for wanting to go to medical school. This needs to be the best personal statement you've ever written; and that means spending lots of time editing and proofreading, as well as having others read it.

Section 9: Standardized Tests. In this section, you'll include the MCAT exams you've taken or are scheduled to take. Many schools will not accept scores that are more than 3 years old. When you take the MCAT, scores are automatically released to AMCAS unless you void your score at the time of the exam. Releasing your scores means that you cannot unrelease them, and they'll be included in your AMCAS application. This section also includes other tests such as the GRE if you want to include those scores as well.

Once you've completed, made changes, and carefully reviewed all the sections, you'll have to certify the AMCAS application. This is as binding as a legal signature. Only certain parts of the application can be changed, so make certain that you go over each section several times before submitting. The changes allowed are:

- ID numbers
- Name
- Contact information
- Date of birth, address, and sex
- Additions to letters of evaluation
- Next MCAT test date
- Additional medical schools
- Release application to premedical advisor

When you're done, you select your payment method, click continue, and hope that the verification process goes smoothly. If, after verification, you notice that there's a problem with AMCAS not calculating your GPAs properly, you have 10 days to petition and try to get the issue resolved. This is not likely, but in some cases a correction can mean a few points added to your GPA and could mean the difference between an interview or not.

If you submit early, and there are no glitches, your application should be processed quickly. Check your application status regularly, since AMCAS is not responsible. If a medical school doesn't receive your materials within 2 to 4 weeks after AMCAS has processed the application, you must notify AMCAS and let them know. If, for any reason, you withdraw your application, you can no longer apply to medical schools that year and your processing fee will not be refunded.

A medical school does not know how many other medical schools you've applied to, so you don't have to worry about anyone knowing that information. However, beginning in February of the application cycle, schools will be able to see how many acceptances you have and your acceptance action. Then, beginning April 1 of the application cycle, medical schools have access to a list of all applicants with a current acceptance action.

After your application is verified, it's sent to your designated medical schools. In a few weeks, you'll begin to receive secondary applications that require additional information and usually another essay. These will also require a fee. Once you complete those and send them off, any interested medical school will contact you for interviews. That's a good indication that your chances for admission are good.

New Sections in the 2025 AMCAS Application

Students applying to medical school in 2025 will be completing a newly revised AMCAS application. The new sections added to previous years are and there are:

- **Work/Activities section that includes Social Justice/Advocacy:** Allows applicants to include experience in advancing the rights, privileges, or opportunities of a person, group, or cause.
- **Other Impactful Experiences:** Replaces the self-reporting Disadvantaged Status question with examples of an applicant's lived experiences and challenges.
- **Institutional Action question includes categories for Conduct and Academic:** Explains any disciplinary and/or academic issues during an applicant's undergraduate education.
- **Optional field that indicates an upcoming AAMC PREview® exam registration date:** Allows applicants to indicate intention to take the PREview exam and when medical schools should expect an applicant's score.
- **Pronoun and Gender Identity have been updated:** The "Other" category option has been replaced with "Another Gender Identity" and "Another pronoun set."

Non-AMCAS Participating Medical Schools

All U.S. medical schools except for those located in Texas, and a few others, participate in AMCAS. The Texas schools use the Texas Medical & Dental Schools Application Service or TMDAS. If you plan on applying to any of these schools, contact the admissions office directly and request an application. The non-AMCAS medical schools are:

Baylor College of Medicine

Brown University School of Medicine

Columbia University College of Physicians and Surgeons

Harvard Medical School

Johns Hopkins University School of Medicine

New York University School of Medicine

Texas A&M University College of Medicine

Texas Tech University Health Science Center School of Medicine

University of Missouri-Kansas City School of Medicine

University of North Dakota School of Medicine

University of Texas Southwestern Medical Center at Dallas Southwestern Medical School

University of Texas Medical School at Galveston

University of Texas School of Medicine at Houston

University of Texas School of Medicine at San Antonio

Yale University School of Medicine

If your plan is to apply to both AMCAS and non-AMCAS participating schools, start early enough so that you have plenty of time to complete both applications. Some students have a hard-enough time working on one application much less having to work on two different ones. My suggestion is to look over both applications months ahead of time so that you're comfortable with the process and have sufficient time to get all your materials submitted for review. Also, make sure you have all the application deadlines written down and posted, since no medical school will accept late applications.

Choosing a New Versus Established Medical School

Because of the need for more doctors, several new medical schools have opened, with more scheduled to be opened within the next few years. The question many potential applicants ask is, "Should I consider one of these newer schools or only apply to the more established programs?" The answer depends on your qualifications and your future goals. Here are some things to consider in making that decision:

- **New medical schools typically have smaller class sizes**. Until a medical program becomes more established, it usually has smaller class sizes. This is a concern for some students who may feel there wouldn't be a large enough network of other students for study and collaboration. On the other hand, if small is better for you, and you think you would like a more intimate environment, with smaller classes and fewer faculty, then a new medical school may work for you.
- **Applicants to newer schools typically have lower grades and MCAT scores**. If you don't have strong qualifications or your grades and MCAT scores are not as competitive as many other applicants, then a newer medical school might take a chance on you. Since they don't get as many applications, and the ones they do get are usually not as strong, your chances are probably better than they otherwise would be.
- **Graduates from new medical schools may not get as many residency spots**. Older, more established medical programs are more prestigious than ones at younger schools, so naturally they would place more of their graduates in residencies. And because the number of medical students is going to outpace the growth of residency slots, students graduating from newer medical schools will face more competition.
- **New medical schools may not have a strong relationship with local hospitals**. One of the important questions to ask is whether a medical school has a relationship with the hospitals at which students will do their rotations. In most cases, they do, but applicants need to make sure that physicians at local hospitals will continually work with students. Clinical rotations are important to a student's education, and the weeks spent learning about a specialty is critical. So before applying to a newer

school, insist on knowing how involved the local hospitals are with medical students.

- **New medical schools may not have as many specialty resources**. If you know what specialties interest you, then you need to ask if the medical school has the resources or the department for you to rotate through. For example, if your interest is plastic surgery but the new medical school does not have the resources in that specialty, then the school is probably not a good fit for you.
- **New medical schools might focus more on primary care**. The trend over the next decade is primary care. Some established medical schools are already trying to attract students who are interested in that field, but many of the newer schools are especially interested in applicants who can convince them that primary care is what they want to do. If that is your interest, then a new medical school may very well fit the bill. This is especially true if your qualifications are not especially strong, but your extracurricular activities indicate that you're a good candidate for primary care.

Fifteen Recently Established Medical Schools

Between 2010 and 2018, fifteen new medical schools opened their doors. These newer schools, which have not established a long-term reputation like some of the older and more traditional schools, may offer a better chance for admission. The following is a list of the schools in the order they were accredited:

Medical School	State	Est.	First Class
Central Michigan University College of Medicine	MI	2012	2016
Frank H. Netter MD School of Medicine at Quinnipiac University	CT	2012	2016
University of California Riverside School of Medicine	CA	2012	2016
University of South Carolina – Greenville School of Medicine	SC	2012	2016
Western Michigan University Howard Stryker MD School of Medicine	MI	2012	2016
University of Texas Rio Grande Valley School of Medicine	TX	2013	2017
California Northstate University College of Medicine	CA	2015	2019
College of Henricopolis School of Medicine	VA	2016	2020
CUNY School of Medicine	NY	2016	2020

Mayo Medical School	AZ	2016	2020
University of Texas at Austin School of Medicine	TX	2016	2020
Indiana University School of Medicine - Evansville	IN	2017	2021
Roseman University of Health Sciences College of Medicine	NV	2017	2021
Seton Hall University School of Medicine	NJ	2017	2021
Washington State University School of Medicine	WA	2017	2021

Newest Accredited Medical Schools (2018 – 2025)

The most recently accredited medical schools sometimes have difficulty recruiting a large enough pool of candidates. There's a perception by some applicants that the newest medical schools may not be as good academically, or may not offer the same advantages when it comes to getting residencies after graduation. So here's an opportunity to apply to schools that might be looking outside the box, so to speak, and will be accepting students who may not be as successful when applying to older, more established programs. The following are sixteen schools that have accepted incoming applicants in the last six years or that will be opening by 2025:

Medical School	State	Est.	First Class
NOVA Southeastern University College of Medicine	FL	2018	2022
California University of Science & Medicine School of Medicine	CA	2018	2022
Carle Illinois College of Medicine	IL	2018	2022
Hackensack Meridian School of Medicine	NJ	2018	2022
TCU & UNTHSC School of Medicine	TX	2018	2022
Anne Burnett Marion School of Medicine at TCU	TX	2019	2023
NYU Long Island School of Medicine (3-year medical school)	NY	2019	2023
Kaiser Permanente School of Medicine	CA	2020	2024
University of Houston, Tilman J. Fertitta Family College of Medicine	TX	2020	2024

University of California, Merced School of Medicine	CA	2023	2027
University of Texas, Tyler School of Medicine	TX	2023	2027
Charles Drew University of Medicine & Science	CA	2024	2028
Duquesne University College of Medicine	PA	2024	2028
Wake Forest University, Charlotte Campus School of Medicine	NC	2024	2028
Thomas F. Frist, Jr. College of Medicine	TN	2025	2029
Alice L. Walton School of Medicine	AR	2025	2029
Xavier University College of Medicine (HBCU)	LA	2025	2029

How Many Applications to Submit

There are different reasons students choose certain medical schools. Some have programs you may be interested in, others offer research opportunities or are in great locations. But most students choose several medical schools because the odds are better. After all, what are the chances that you'll get accepted to Harvard if that's your only choice compared to your chances of getting accepted to one of fifteen medical schools you apply to?

Although the number of schools you apply to improve your odds, it won't matter much if your credentials are poor. You can apply to 25 medical schools, but if you have a 2.0 GPA and low MCAT scores, you won't get accepted to any of them. However, if only one of your qualifications is below par, and you can explain that discrepancy, then a few medical schools might see you as a potential candidate for their program.

When applying to medical schools, be realistic in your self-evaluation, but never feel you shouldn't apply to a medical school just because your credentials are not outstanding. I've helped several students with average GPAs get into medical school because they had other exceptional qualifications. In 2024, the average number of applications was 18, which means that some students submitted many more than that. Before submitting too many applications, consider three things:

1. **The cost.** Besides the initial AMCAS processing fee, there's a fee for each additional medical school you apply to. After that expense, each medical school will then send you a secondary application, which typically costs more than the additional fees that AMCAS charges for applying to multiple schools. In the end, you might be paying upwards of $1,000 depending on how many schools you've applied to and how many secondary applications you send back.
2. **The time involved.** Completing and submitting the AMCAS application is just the beginning. A few weeks after verification, you'll be receiving secondary applications that include more information and more essays. The more secondary applications

you receive, the more time you will have to spend working on them. And if time is a factor in your life, consider the number of schools you apply to. Anything over 20 schools and you're going to have a difficult time submitting quality secondaries.

3. **Your grades and MCAT scores.** No matter what the new trends in medical school admission and education are, the two most important factors admission committees consider will always be grades and MCAT scores. It doesn't matter if you're the most compassionate and caring person in the world if you're not going to make it through a rigorous curriculum and pass the medical boards. In the past decade, successful applicants have had GPAs between 3.5 and 4.0 and MCAT scores above 510. The new MCAT's scoring is different than it was in the past; and although it's still too early to predict how the new MCAT scores will affect success on medical school boards, it's safe to say that successful applicants should strive for an overall total score of 510 or above. A score of 528 means that the student is in the 99th percentile of all test takers. A score of 472 places the student at the bottom or in the bottom one percent of test takers. In 2023-24, the average GPA was 3.75 and the average MCAT score was 512.

When it comes to deciding how many schools to apply to, or whether or not you're an excellent candidate who will have no problem getting accepted, there's a good rule of thumb regarding grades and MCAT scores. The following table illustrates the range of qualifications and what's considered acceptable when considering GPA and both old and new versions of the MCAT. We probably won't have good statistics on the new MCAT until 2025, but again, we can assume that a good score on the new MCAT is 510 or above.

Student Rating	GPA	Old MCAT Scores	New MCAT Scores
Excellent	3.7 – 4.0	35 – 45	516 - 528
Very Good	3.4 – 3.69	30 – 34	511 - 515
Average	3.0 – 3.39	25 – 29	500 - 510
Below Average	2.8 – 2.99	20 – 24	490 - 499
Poor	2.0 – 2.79	5 – 19	472 - 489

In some cases, low MCAT scores, if they're not too low, can be overcome with high grades, especially in science courses. However, a school may look at high grades and low MCAT scores as an indication of grade inflation or a weak premed program. On the other hand, high MCAT scores and average grades may indicate intelligence but either a poor work ethic or some hardship a student had to face that affected his or her grades. In any case, the ratings above are not hard and fast rules, and that's why admissions committee members rely on other factors as well.

Two factors that could place you in the excellent category would be a record of exceptional extracurricular activities, especially in research or a health-related field, and outstanding letters of recommendation. Because of that, don't hesitate to apply to certain medical schools just because you don't think they would find you competitive. At the same time, be realistic about your chances of admission to out-of-state or some of the nation's most prestigious medical schools. Unless you're exceptional in every other way, you're not going to be successful applying to John's Hopkins with a 3.0 GPA, or to out-of-state schools that only accept a high percentage of in-state residents.

Because the average number of applications per student is 18, admission statistics and acceptance rates can be deceiving. For example, at one medical school, 125 students were enrolled, even though almost 300 acceptances were offered. At another private medical school, 200 students were enrolled but almost 400 were accepted. The other students chose to enter other programs, or they delayed their plans until the following year. So when you look at the percent of student enrollments at medical schools, keep in mind that a school must accept more students than it can handle to fill the allotted class space. This means that instead of having a 1 in 5 chance of getting accepted, a good student has a 1 in 2 chance if he or she chooses medical schools that are good bets for success.

After you've assessed your credentials and your chances for admission to both in-state and national schools, decide on your list. Be selective, optimistic, and realistic. I knew one student who applied to 21 medical schools and didn't get accepted to any, but I also knew a student who was accepted to all 4 schools on her list because she was very selective in which schools she applied to. Less prestigious schools, competing against better known schools, often accept as many as 60 percent of the applicants to fill their quotas. Chances for admission, therefore, become much better if you plan your applications properly and if you're wise enough to apply to a wide range of medical schools. Your chances depend entirely on your credentials (GPA and MCAT), your qualifications, your letters of recommendation, and how you present yourself on the interview. It's a numbers game. But it's a game you can win if you're persistent and you plan accordingly.

Reapplying to Medical School

According to admissions committee members I'd spoken to, it's a good idea to reapply to medical school several times if you're not accepted on the first try. Over the years, I've helped many students overcome some of their shortcomings and improve their chances of success two and sometimes three years later. One committee member even suggested that if a student is serious about being a physician, he or she might consider reapplying four years in a row. There are several reasons for this:

1. Schools periodically change deans of admission, who have their own set of criteria and standards for determining borderline cases. Admissions committee members also change and may look at your qualifications and/or credentials in an entirely different light. This could mean the difference between outright rejection and being

waitlisted (placed on hold for possible admission).

2. In any given year, for whatever reason, a student's application may not be examined as thoroughly as it should be. One case I was told about involved a delay in the application screening process. When it was time to look at the mound of applications, the committee made quick judgments and probably eliminated some students who might otherwise have gotten more consideration.
3. There's an entirely new pool of applicants each year with different backgrounds, credentials, and qualifications. Placing yourself with a new applicant pool can certainly affect your standing, often for the better, especially if you've worked on your weaknesses during that year.
4. Applicants who reapply several times are viewed as serious about wanting to go to medical school. The time and effort required to apply and then reapply several times is substantial. By showing perseverance, while continuing to improve your credentials and doing volunteer work, you'll demonstrate to admissions committees that you're the kind of individual who would do well in medical school.

Being rejected by medical schools doesn't have to be the end of the road. I've known students who had tried time and again before finally getting accepted because they stuck it out, but especially because they continued to work on building their credentials. Admissions committees cannot help but look favorably on someone so determined to become a doctor that he or she will keep improving in order to be accepted. Often, an extra year of work in one area is all that's needed. So, rather than rush off to a foreign medical school, or give up altogether, try a few more times. If you're serious about medicine, your desire will show through and your chances for admission will improve markedly.

Women Applicants

Over the years, the number of women applying to and being accepted to medical schools has grown tremendously. In fact, 2023-24 was the fifth year in a row that women made up the majority of applicants and matriculants. The following table shows a significant trend in women being accepted to medical school beginning in 1950. In 2003, the number of women applicants had outnumbered men for the first time in history, with 50.8 percent of the total applicant pool that year being women. In 2024-2025, the percentage of women accepted to medical schools was 55%.

Year	Total Women Applicants	Number Accepted
1950-1951	1390	385
1960-1961	1026	600
1970-1971	2289	1297

1980-1981	10644	4970
1990-1991	13,462	5,866
2008-2009	20,360	9,181
2010-2011	20,207	9,237
2014-2015	23,019	10,194
2016-2017	25,600	10,940
2020-2021	28,343	12,417
2022-2023	31,190	13,268
2024-2025	29,763	12,758

In the past, attracting women was difficult because most women didn't take the science and math courses required for admission. Today, however, there are as many women in math and science classes as there are men. Also, admissions committees in the past were set on your typical "science types," whereas today's medical schools are just as willing to accept non-science majors, as long as they complete the required courses for admission and are equally as qualified. Moreover, women have proven themselves to be excellent medical students and doctors, shattering old beliefs that a medical career is too rigorous. So, regardless of what you think your chances for admission are, don't let anything stop you from applying, if medicine is really what you want to do.

Age and the Applicant

How old is too old? Will medical schools question why you're only now deciding to go to medical school? Is there a certain cut off age? These are some of the questions older applicants ask as they decide whether to take the plunge. Being an older applicant definitely has its challenges because different schools have different criteria regarding age limits. Legally, a medical school cannot discriminate based on age, but a medical school faculty member told me that if an admissions committee member wants to keep you out, they can do so easily and make it look as if age had nothing to do with it. Until recently, it was unheard of to find a medical student over the age of 35. The good news is that the average age of incoming students has increased over the years and is now closer to 24.

Several sources have told me that the "unofficial" age limit for most medical schools is indeed 35. This assumes that a person that age, if he or she finishes 4 years of medical school and 3 to 6 years of residency, can still practice medicine for at least 20 years after that. Training a physician takes a lot of time and money, so naturally medical schools would like their graduates to contribute as many years to practicing medicine as they can.

One committee member I'd spoken to said that more medical schools are looking at older applicants in a new light and with more flexibility that they ever had in the past. And because society is beginning to downplay age as a social issue – even accepting the fact that older individuals often make better and more conscientious students – medical schools are changing their thinking to reflect the views of society in general. In fact, some years ago, a 51-year old woman graduated from UCLA School of Medicine, the oldest graduate in that school's history.

With the population aging, and with more students waiting to go to college, incoming freshman have more diverse backgrounds and experiences than ever before. By the time they graduate, they're not typical 21-year olds. They're viewed as more mature, stable, and experienced, qualities considered essential during medical school training. However, these older applicants need to be prepared to defend their decision much more vigorously than younger applicants. Before going on interviews, older applicants should review all the positive aspects of their age and use that to their advantage. If they don't, interviewers will use that against them in their final evaluations.

The trend for acceptance of older applicants looks good. While only 12 percent of applicants age 30 and older were admitted in 1978, almost 25 percent were admitted by 2015. According to Jay Bryde, Admissions Officer at Michigan State, "Our classes typically have several students in their 30s, an occasional student in their 40s, and rarely a student older than that." He believes that non-traditional applicants bring maturity and life experiences to the classroom. To convince admissions committee members you have what it takes, here are suggestions for the personal statement that will make age work for you.

- **Address why you're embarking on a medical career now.** There will be questions about why you're giving up your current career and choosing years of medical training. You must address why you want to change careers, how it will impact your life, especially if you have a family, and how you came to this decision later in life. You must also address concerns about how personal responsibilities might distract you from medical studies. Avoid being negative about your employer or career, Instead focus on the events in your life that finally made you decide on a career in medicine.
- **Be specific about your strengths and experiences.** As an older individual, you have the benefit of maturity and experience. You also have skills that younger students do not, and you've certainly demonstrated your ability to work hard and overcome obstacles in life. No matter what you've done, highlight the things that you'll bring to medical school and that will benefit other students as well.
- **Convince the committee that you're serious and motivated about medicine.** More so than with younger applicants, admission committee members will want to make certain that you're serious. If you've continued to do volunteer work in the medical field, you'll show the admissions committee you have what it takes. Use your

firsthand experiences to illustrate your desire and your ability to succeed at all costs.

One final note on age and the applicant is that age can be used to your advantage if you've participated in other non-academic activities. Work, volunteer services, leadership positions, and involvement in community organizations all show a willingness to become engaged. In essence, you'll be demonstrating a proven track record critical for medical school, something a younger individual may not have. So don't think for a moment that age will hinder your chances for admission. With a little planning and foresight, you can turn your age into a positive attribute that will make admissions committees choose you, not despite your age but because of it.

Letters of Recommendation

Depending on the medical school, you'll need to supply 2-3 letters of recommendation from individuals who know you well or from the premedical advisory committee at your undergraduate institution. More and more medical schools are beginning to require a composite letter from a premedical evaluation committee (if there is one at your college or university) rather than individual letters. If your college has such a committee, but the medical school you're applying to will accept letters from either individuals or from a committee, choose the committee. A medical school, naturally, would prefer a letter from an evaluations committee, and it would not look favorably on your part to opt for individual letters in that case. When discussing letters with committee members, don't hesitate to ask them if there's any information they need from you in order to help them draft it.

Letters are valuable to admissions committees because they can offer the committee members an insight into your character and personality they may not otherwise detect from your application. For this reason, make every effort to become available and familiar to your advisory committee members without becoming a nuisance. I've seen students try so hard to get noticed by premedical faculty that they present a negative image. Don't be obnoxious. The best way to get to know faculty members is to participate in activities where faculty members will notice you and to pay them an occasional visit at an appropriate time (designated office hours) in order to discuss your plans and ask their advice. If a medical school or your premedical advisory committee requires letters from individuals, there are a few suggestions you should follow to make the best impression possible.

- Make sure you know the person well before asking for a letter of recommendation. A friend of mine was rejected by a genetic counseling firm even though she was intelligent, personable, and well-qualified because of a bad letter of recommendation. Apparently, the person writing the letter commented that she seemed immature and disagreeable. She learned the hard way that asking for a letter doesn't necessarily flatter someone into writing nice things. Be careful and be very selective.

- Make sure that the individual writing the letter knows your background, character, personality, and motivation, and would be willing to tell the admissions committee about the qualities you have that would make you a good physician. That's why letters from physicians you've shadowed are so effective. It's a waste of time to have someone who doesn't know you write a letter. When a student I've seen only once or twice asks me for a letter of recommendation, I'll either refuse to do it or I'll write a general letter in which I actually say that I don't know this person all that well. Not a good reflection on you, as far as admissions committees go. A general rule of thumb is to get to know a faculty member well enough that he or she knows you by name.
- Explain to the person writing the letter what specific medical schools are looking for in terms of qualifications, character, personal qualities, etc. Most individuals, especially if they're non-science types, are not familiar with medical school admissions criteria. Be honest and specify the kinds of things that an effective medical school letter should contain. Here are some particularly important characteristics to include:

  Personal Attributes: Discuss how the applicant interacts with others. Specify special characteristics that make the applicant suited for the study of medicine. Emphasize why the student has promise or potential for medicine. Use specific examples if possible rather than generalities.

  Academic Achievement: Without mentioning specific grades, emphasize why the student is capable of high academic achievement. Mention course difficulty, class standing, heavy course loads while participating in extracurricular activities and/or work programs, student teaching, honors and awards, increasingly better GPA during upper level courses, etc.

  Overall Impressions and Evaluation: At the conclusion of the letter, a concise summary paragraph should contain a value judgment about the student's main strengths and why he or she would be an excellent candidate for medical school.

- Don't ask teachers, whose only contact with you has been a class or two, to send letters. Admissions committee members can see for themselves whether you're a good student from your transcripts. They don't need to plod through a superficial letter by someone who hardly knows you outside of class. Sometimes, the winning quality an admissions committee is looking for is reflected by an individual who knows your personality well. If letters are to be sent by individuals, here are some good sources:
  - ❑ Supervisor or boss who can tell first-hand about your motivation, work ethic, maturity, and dependability. A well-written letter from someone who will detail how intelligent and hard-working you are will always trump an impersonal letter, even if it's from someone famous.
  - ❑ A respected professional such as a doctor, lawyer, banker, etc. The best letter is from a physician who you have spent time with.

- ❑ Directors who are personally familiar with your volunteer activities in hospitals, clinics, and other healthcare settings.
- ❑ Faculty members who know you well or who you've done research projects with.

There are rules for asking someone for a letter of recommendation. First, don't be presumptuous or arrogant about it. After all, they're going out of their way by doing this for you, so make sure you're polite, but also make sure they know how important this is. Ask them if they can **honestly and without reservation** give you a **positive** letter that includes the types of characteristics mentioned. Offer to give them a resume that lists your schooling, major accomplishments, work and volunteer history, etc. This way, the writer can personalize the letter of recommendation and make it more genuine and interesting.

At some schools, premed students have a choice of having information such as letters in a file that's either open or closed to them. Given the choice, always select the closed file since admissions committees know that writers will be less likely to be honest and write something negative if they know the student has access to the file. Some medical schools require that you have a closed file so the information is more unbiased.

Most medical schools rely on letters of recommendation as one of the last criteria in making their selections. Sometimes, letters can be the deciding factor. It would be terrible if you failed to gain admission to medical school because you asked the wrong person to write a letter. Personal friends, family members, and co-workers should never write letters for you! Therefore, the three most important factors to consider are: (1) know the person well enough that he or she will write a strong, positive, and honest letter, (2) be selective in who writes the letter, with the best letters being from physicians you've shadowed or directors of places in which you'd volunteered, and (3) get to know the premedical faculty and advisory committee at your college very well so that they know you personally and will vouch for your achievements and activities.

The Personal Statement

Section 8 of the AMCAS application is the personal essay section, and is designed to help you explain why you've selected medicine as a career, what motivates you, what medical schools should know about you that hasn't been discussed in other parts of the application, what hardships, challenges, and obstacles you've encountered, and reasons why your academic record may have suffered at some point in your life. AMCAS gives you room for one, single-spaced page or about 5,300 characters. After reading your essay, admissions committee members must be able to answer three questions: Why does the applicant want to be a doctor? What experiences has she had that led to that decision? What has the applicant done to cultivate her interest in being a physician?

Use every line you possibly can, otherwise the admissions committee will assume that you either: 1) lack significant experiences in your life, 2) haven't learned much in your life, 3) don't care enough to write about what you've experienced, or 4) think that your application is so good that you don't need to write very much in the personal comments section. This is a serious mistake! Fill the entire page. One medical school admissions officer revealed that applicants who have good GPA/MCAT scores are rejected every year based on poorly written essays. He made the analogy that "Neglecting to write a strong personal statement is like heading out on a long automobile trip and draining the oil out of your engine. You're just not going to get far even if your engine appeared to be in great shape. You need to have a well-written and coherent personal statement."

Read and reread your statement several times, making changes and corrections as needed. Put it aside for a few days and then come back to it again with fresh ideas and a better way to phrase sentences. Going back to your work after not seeing it will make editing easier. Mistakes will leap off the page at you, and you'll remember things you may not have thought of during the first or second draft.

As you rewrite your essay, emphasize key accomplishments and, without being too obnoxious, don't be too modest. Your essay is one of hundreds, if not thousands, seen by admissions committees, and it needs to stand out. I can't emphasize enough how much this area of the selection process could mean and how you should do everything you can to ensure that, after reading your essay, an admissions committee will be convinced of your potential as a medical student. Your goal is to clinch that all important interview.

Once you've written several drafts, it's a good idea to have your premed advisor and/or an English major read and edit it for grammatical errors. A blatant error can make the most understanding committee member have second thoughts. You don't want to ruin an otherwise good application at this point. Here are some suggestions that will help you write the best personal statement you can:

- **Begin with a strong opening.** Admissions committees consist of both faculty and students who try to create a diverse student body with various backgrounds. Grab their attention right away with a catchy opening that demonstrates why you would be a great addition to their program. Think about what makes your personal story special and unique. Avoid at all costs the "I want to help people" or "I want to make a difference" lines. Admissions officers have heard those a thousand times.
- **Center your essay on a main theme.** Think about the main event or experience in your life that influenced your decision to go into medicine. Weave that theme throughout the essay so that the admissions committee members get a sense of why you would make a good physician.
- **Emphasize the personal qualities that will make you a good doctor.** Central to your application are the questions, "Why do I want to be a doctor?" and "Why should medical schools select me?" Tell the committee that you know how challenging a medical education will be, how much commitment and dedication is involved, what your passions are, what life experiences you've had that led you to this decision, and what qualities you possess that will make you succeed. Highlight your strengths; and make your background and what shaped you as a person set you apart.
- **Demonstrate enthusiasm.** Show the admissions committees that you're enthusiastic about medicine by including work-related experiences that have stimulated your

interest in being a doctor and contributed to your growth as a human being. Narrow your focus to one or two main themes or relevant experiences rather than a laundry list of accomplishments.

- **Demonstrate knowledge of the medical field.** Admissions committees need to know you're serious about a medical career. When you include information about your knowledge of medicine, be specific and use language which conveys that knowledge, books you've read, or people you talked to that have helped your decision.
- **Don't duplicate what's already on your AMCAS application.** Skip the mentions of GPA, courses you've taken, etc. The personal statement should be distinctive and a means of detailing parts of your history the admissions committee doesn't know about. A detailed anecdote of something that influenced your decision is always a good strategy. However, don't gloss over any potential red flags like a few low science grades. Make sure you address why this happened and how you've overcome any hardships since then.
- **Don't generalize.** Simply stating that you would be a great doctor is not enough. Be specific. Convince the committee by including concrete examples and specific experiences that will back up your claim. However, avoid examples from your high school years, and never include your personal political or religious views. No one cares, and it might detract from your application.
- **Don't exaggerate.** According to a recent survey, more than 80 percent of medical school admissions officers reported that claims made by some applicants were either false or exaggerated. Nothing is worse than getting as far as the interview, only to get tripped up because you lied or exaggerated on the personal statement. Integrity is especially important. If you have so few life experiences that you must misrepresent yourself, you probably need to reevaluate your decision to apply in the first place.
- **Avoid the dreaded essay mistakes.** Never mention the following: money as a motivating factor, clichés and trite statements, quotes by someone else, opinions that seem like preaching, gimmicky language and style, arrogance and self-praise, political or religious statements.
- **Be concise.** A one-page personal statement is the rule, so make sure it's concise, edited, and interesting. Always have a few other people proofread it, and then revise, rewrite, and rewrite again until it's perfect. Use the computer spell check, use a thesaurus to avoid duplicating words, and finally ask an English teacher or English major to read it and offer suggestions about grammar, syntax, punctuation, and style.

Never underestimate the importance of the personal statement. The decision to grant an applicant an interview is sometimes based on the contents of his or her essay. If you're a borderline student, give your statement the attention it deserves. Be serious about it; never write anything humorous or clever. Your aim is to ensure that it stands out compared with the others. A friend of mine, who has interviewed numerous medical school candidates, had the following to say about the personal statement:

"When I read a personal statement, what I don't want to see is a long exposé about why the student wants to become a doctor. I want to read about his or her accomplishments. After all, a 22-year-old has no real experience in medicine, so I don't care to read about medicine. I want to see whether that person is caring, motivated, an independent thinker, and inspires others to act. Medicine is a very heavy pressure career, and a person who chooses medicine must have demonstrated the ability to make decisions, be independent, and assume a good deal of responsibility. Those are the qualities that need to shine through on the statement.

One essay I remember well was written by a student who oversaw a school cafeteria. He supervised 60 students and was responsible for scheduling work assignments and vacations and had to make sure that everyone knew what to do during the workday. When I interviewed him several months later, we spent most of the time talking about his work at the cafeteria. I knew from his essay and the ensuing interview that, even though he didn't have any experience in medicine, he would make a fantastic doctor."

When you're writing your personal statement, don't make the mistake of thinking that what you consider insignificant accomplishments don't mean much to admissions committee members. They can mean the difference between acceptance and rejection. If you've done anything showing you to be a creative, take-charge, responsible person who inspires others to accomplish goals, include that in your essay. Any committee member who reads about a person like that would no doubt take notice and say, "Hey, medicine could use someone like that." In a survey conducted by the American Medical Association, 60 percent of medical schools used the personal statement to evaluate an applicant's motivation, maturity, compassion, leadership, and integrity. That's how important it is.

Sample Personal Essay

The following is a personal statement written by an applicant who is now a successful pediatrician. It includes many of the criteria important in grabbing a reader's attention and holding his or her interest.

Born in Jefferson, North Carolina, I was raised with two younger sisters and a younger brother. My grandfather owns a farm; and my father, being an only son, took over the farm after my grandfather suffered a stroke nearly five years ago. Even before that incident, though, I had always been involved in farm work, mostly tending cattle and growing corn. For the past three years, I've also been in charge of taking care of more than 4,000 Christmas trees, which takes up much of my time while I'm at home. I think of my trees more as a hobby than a chore, since I really enjoy the opportunity of being out by myself on a piece of farm I consider my very own.

Because of my closeness with my family, and my responsibilities to the farm, I try to go home nearly every weekend. Until recently, I have been the only pianist at my church, and am depended upon to be there every Sunday. My two sisters and my brother, who I try to see as much as possible, also give me an added reason for visiting often. My grandfather, now in a wheelchair because of his stroke, still has his car and only gets to ride in it when I'm there to drive him.

In making my decision to apply to medical school, I have constantly debated about what is required of a doctor, and whether this is a career for me. I have always thought of a doctor as both a scientist and a social worker, two professions that I've always had a desire to pursue. Socially, I have always been active in my community and my church. Being the leader of my youth group, I've worked closely with my pastor in planning county-wide youth events and visiting the sick and needy, especially during Christmas.

I have worked many different jobs, always learning to deal with a different group of people. Working as a pharmacy drug clerk in the lower working-class section of Winston-Salem has given me confidence that I have the ability to deal with sick and often frightened people. My volunteer work at North Carolina Baptist Hospital has also given me an insight into what caring for the sick and dying is all about. When dealing with and caring for my grandfather, I had to show both strength and compassion because the attitude I had toward him would have determined how he looked and how he felt about his handicap. If there is one personal quality that I would extend to my work as a doctor, it would be my willingness to touch the lives of my patients in a sincere and humane way. I think that it's essential for a doctor to deal with people on a one-on-one basis, and my work has given me the opportunity to learn just that.

Love of science has also affected my decision to apply to medical school. After being a volunteer in surgery research at Wake Forest University School of Medicine, I decided to do undergraduate research in chemistry. I soon found out that success, and sometimes failure, are part of the learning process, and that we all need to accept our failures to become more successful and better human beings.

In thinking about a medical career, I've come to realize that there's an increasing need for doctors who are willing to serve small town hospital and rural communities. I also realize that the reward for serving these hospitals and communities is not so much financial as it is a personal satisfaction. Knowing this has not discouraged me from my principle goal: to serve those communities and their people in the best way I possibly can, as a family physician in a rural community.

WWAMI and WICHE Programs

WWAMI is a program that accepts students from Washington, Wyoming, Alaska, Montana, and Idaho. Each participating state admits a specific number of medical students each year who are supported through tuition assistance covering the full cost of medical education. Students spend their first year at state universities in their home states: University of Alaska (Anchorage), Montana State University, University of Idaho, and University of Wyoming. The second year of the program is spent at the University of Washington School of Medicine in Seattle, after which students have the opportunity to complete their third- and fourth-year clerkships throughout the WWAMI states.

WICHE is the acronym for Western Interstate Commission for Higher Education. It's a regional, nonprofit organization that includes the 15 western states of Alaska, Arizona, California, Colorado, Hawaii, Idaho, Montana, Nevada, New Mexico, North and South Dakota, Oregon, Utah, Washington, Wyoming, and the U.S. Pacific Territories. These member states work to improve access to higher education and ensure student success through exchange programs and regional initiatives.

Fee Assistance Program (FAP)

The AAMC helps to defray some of the costs of applying to medical school by offering financial assistance to qualified AMCAS applicants. Benefits include:

- Reduced MCAT registration and rescheduling fees.
- AMCAS application fee waiver.
- Official Guide to the MCAT Exam (e-book), and online practice questions.
- MCAT sample test and practice question sets.
- Access to the Medical School Admission Requirements database.

Most AMCAS-participating medical schools waive any supplemental application fees.

Applying for Residence Status

If you're serious about medical school but don't have the qualifications to compete against better students, one alternative is to become a resident of a state with many medical schools. This would help your chances since most applicants come from the state in which the medical school is located. Here are some reasons for applying for state residency:

- You would join a statewide applicant pool that, in general, is probably not as academically well-qualified as you would be. Normally, the out-of-state applicant pools have higher GPAs and MCAT scores than in-state applicant pools.
- You will increase your chances of acceptance from 1 in 100 to 1 in 3 in some cases.
- Employment for one year is a good life experience to include on your application.
- The medical school will see you as someone who's serious enough about medical school to be willing to relocate to gain admission.

To become a legal resident, you must show that you came to that state with the true intention of becoming a legal resident. Residency requirements vary from state to state, but you would probably be assured legal resident status if you do the following:

1. Get a job in that state
2. File income tax as a state resident
3. Get a state driver's license and registration
4. Register to vote
5. Open a savings and checking account
6. Purchase property

7. Establish credit within the state by opening charge accounts

The timeline at the beginning of the chapter should help you chart your course for preparing for and applying to medical school. If you're serious about getting admitted to medical school, visit your premed advisor regularly and review the timetable every semester so that you stay on track. This will help you avoid the common pitfalls like not scheduling classes properly, not allowing enough time to study for the MCAT, not taking the MCAT in time, missing deadlines, or making mistakes on the AMCAS application. Starting your very first semester, and being diligent about schoolwork and volunteer activities, will greatly enhance your chances of being successful.

CHAPTER 5

THE ADMISSIONS PROCESS

Twenty years ago, a 3.75 GPA and stellar MCAT scores would just about guarantee admission to medical school. The nation's top schools would compete over valedictorians and exceptional students whose resumes included work in research labs and who published journal articles. Volunteer work was great, but as long as you had the grades and graduated from a select college, you were a top contender. And if you happened to have had some good extracurricular activities in addition, then you stood head and shoulders above the rest. On the interview, you would meet with a faculty member or two, answer questions to make sure you were stable, and tour the school.

Today's admission process looks very different. Even though undergraduate GPAs and MCAT scores have been increasing, today's medical school applicant needs more than just a good academic record; he or she needs personality, communication skills, an ability to think critically, and a desire to cooperate and interact with others in a way that enhances the lives of patients. It's an entirely new way of selecting applicants for a twenty-first century medical education. This chapter explains what admissions committees are looking for once they get their hands on your AMCAS application.

AMCAS and Initial Screening of Applicants

Most schools use AMCAS applications for their initial screening. Students whose applications suggest they would have trouble handling a medical school curriculum or whose qualifications are not up to par are rejected. All other applicants are sent an additional supplementary application packet with information regarding other requirements such as letters of evaluation, additional fees, etc. These extra items must be sent directly to the medical school and not to AMCAS.

Because the AMCAS application is often used for initial screening, it's important that you make as good an impression as possible. Don't leave out hardships or disadvantages you faced, and don't be afraid to emphasize your good qualities, since these will be the selling points that may very well award you an interview. You have nothing to lose by marketing your talents and strengths, and everything to gain in terms of successful admission. After all, what good will your efforts and hard work do if no one on the admissions committee knows about them? It's like writing a bestseller and not marketing it.

Never sell yourself short and, above all, don't underestimate the value an admissions committee member will place on your work or activity. What you might think is insignificant, a medical school may consider highly desirable as far as overall preparation for a medical career. This is especially important if your grades or MCAT scores are not as high as they should be. So highlight your experiences, honors, awards, employment, volunteer work, publications, supervisory roles, and military service. Finish the application by completing the personal comments section, which offers a final opportunity for you to sell yourself to the schools you're applying to.

Selection Factors

We can divide the main factors that admissions committees consider into two categories: 1) Objective data and 2) Subjective data. The objective data is academic performance measured by GPA, MCAT scores, an examination of individual transcripts to see the number of courses taken per semester, and how difficult the courses were. The level of difficulty is compared with the amount of preparation the student had taken before taking the course. For example, receiving a C in physics before taking an advanced math class would explain not getting a higher grade. Also considered is whether academic performance had improved, leveled off, or gotten worse. It's never a good sign to see grades dropping.

The subjective data fall into several categories. Non-academic activities such as summer jobs, volunteer work in the medical field, and extracurricular involvement are important. All extra activities, however, are balanced against academic performance. A person who's done nothing but study and get all A's might not be as strong a candidate as the person who had to work twenty hours or more a week to support himself in school, or had spent a good deal of time in community service, and has a B average. Admissions committees also look at special talents and achievements that enable a student to be set apart from the large pool of applicants. Also important are letters of recommendation and how well a student presents him or herself on the interview.

One other subjective factor students seem to overlook is the interest that admissions committees might have in non-traditional fields. Most medical schools are concerned with new disciplines becoming a part of medicine. Social sciences and economics, for example, are becoming increasingly necessary in the health care delivery system. Systems analysts are also going to be important in medicine, as are biomedical engineers, bioethicists, and genetic counselors.

Before applying to medical schools, look at their web sites and read their descriptions and admissions criteria. Some schools place a very heavy emphasis on MCAT scores while other schools do not unless your scores are below average. Most schools won't even consider you if you've never worked or volunteered in a clinical setting. And some schools, especially the big-name research institutions, place an emphasis on research and will not consider applicants that have not had research experience. You wouldn't apply for a job unless you knew what the employer was looking for, would you? The same goes for medical school. By applying to schools that fit well with your background, you'll improve your chances for successful admission.

According to medical school admissions officers, there are certain processes and procedures all medical schools go through when screening applicants. Some schools must contend with thousands of applications a year and pare that number down to the few that will get invited for interviews. Here, from an actual admissions officer, is the process simplified:

Step one: Admissions committee members make sure the applicant has met minimum academic requirements. There's not a better way to make the preliminary cut than to screen by GPA and MCAT scores. If a student doesn't make the preliminary cut, applications are often forwarded to administrative staff that looks for other criteria that may overcome less than stellar grades and MCAT scores. The personal essay, extracurricular activities, and letters of recommendation are important in these cases.

Step two: Age of academic coursework and the number of MCAT attempts is evaluated. If an applicant's transcripts are 10 years ago, for example, and no other current coursework has been taken, admission is highly unlikely. If MCAT scores are more than 3 years old, the applicant would have to retake the exam. Furthermore, if the MCAT was taken multiple times but the scores didn't go up, that's a bad sign. Applicants who take the MCAT more than three times are usually not accepted.

Step three: Applications that make the preliminary cut are sent to admissions committee members who decide if the applicant deserves to be invited for an interview. The criteria for an interview are usually based on three questions: 1) Is the applicant a good fit for the program? 2) Based on the academic transcripts, would the applicant succeed in a demanding curriculum? 3) Would the applicant make a good physician based on the material in the AMCAS application? If the committee members are satisfied, then the applicant is invited for an interview.

Step four: Once the initial review is done, applicants are usually screened again before a rejection letter is sent out. With thousands of applications (some schools may have as many as 10,000), sometimes things get overlooked. One of those is to look at how many hours of coursework an applicant has taken in any given year, as well as the grades earned. For example, if one student took 18 credit hours, including organic chemistry and physics and earned B's, while another student took 10 credit hours but only one science course and got all A's, the first student would be looked at more favorably.

Many interests and disciplines have expanded over the past decade, which continue to add to and contribute to the practice of medicine. And as society becomes increasingly complex, the whole process of medical education and health care delivery will also continue to change. Medical schools no longer admit only the stereotyped premed biology or chemistry major. What this means is that you now have an opportunity to make an impression on admissions committee members if your interests lie in a valuable and needed area of health care. However, remember that a medical school curriculum is grueling, so no matter how much you desire to be a physician, and how good your other qualities are, first and foremost you must be an excellent student with good grades to show for it.

Early Decision Program (EDP)

The early decision program is a way for students to apply to one, and only one, school and receive an admission decision by October 1. The biggest advantage of this program is that you'll already know you've been accepted to a medical school and will not have to worry about applying to multiple schools. One other positive factor is that you'll save time and money by already having been accepted to the medical school of your choice.

Because the early decision program is a binding agreement between the applicant and the medical school, **a student must accept an admission offer**. A student who decides not to accept an offer cannot accept any other offer from any other medical school. Therefore, you need to be sure that the medical school you choose is absolutely the right one for you.

Before submitting an EDP application, read each school's admissions criteria. Some medical schools only accept in-state residents while others accept out-of-state residents only if they apply as EDP applicants. For out-of-state students, the qualifications are high, so only apply if you're an outstanding candidate.

If not accepted to the school of your choice, you will automatically be placed in the regular applicant pool by the school and only then can you apply to other medical schools. Since most of the early decision participating schools admit a small percentage of their class through this program, I would recommend you not apply for early decision unless you have the following minimum qualifications:

- An overall GPA of 3.7 with a science GPA of at least 3.7.
- An overall score of at least 515 on the MCAT.
- An outstanding record of volunteer work and extracurricular activities.
- Excellent letters of evaluation.
- Absolute certainty of the medical school you wish to attend.

Admission Trends for 2025 and Beyond

With rapid changes in medicine and the healthcare system, admissions officers are also changing the way in which they select applicants to medical school. Students graduating from college in 2025 and beyond need to think differently than students did in the past. It's impossible to predict exactly what medical school will be like in the future, but here are some of the trends medical education experts say are happening right now.

- **Competition is increasing**. The number of applicants to U.S. medical schools will be increasing, and that will likely continue well into the future. And with a larger applicant pool comes more competition. Grades and MCAT scores have also been improving, with the average GPA for all applicants nearing 3.80 and average MCAT scores 512. As the number of applicants is soon to approach 60,000, it will be difficult for students with average academic records to be admitted. Recently, when admissions officers were asked about competition, the majority reported that admission will be much more competitive than it was five or ten years ago.

- **Primary care is the future**. An increasing number of medical schools are looking at ways to identify students committed to primary care over higher paying specialties. Over the next decade, medical programs will increase their focus on primary care and, therefore, students who can convince admissions committee members – through their volunteer work at clinics, for example – that they're serious about primary care will gain an advantage in the screening process.
- **Applicants are increasingly selected based on the Holistic Review**. Current and future admissions decisions will include what the AAMC calls the Holistic Review, a flexible, individualized way of assessing an applicant's capabilities based not only on academics but on life experiences, personal attributes, and non-science activities. What schools are looking for are doctors of tomorrow, individuals who can relate to people and who are well-rounded. In fact, in the past few years, U.S. medical schools accepted a greater number of students with undergraduate degrees in Humanities and Social Sciences than ever before.
- **Three-year medical degrees**. As medical education costs increase, and residency programs more difficult to find, more medical schools will offer a three-year medical degree in which courses are condensed so that students can graduate a year earlier. These accelerated programs will be especially valuable in attracting students into choosing primary care. Louisiana State University School of Medicine, New York University School of Medicine and Texas Tech University School of Medicine are the pioneers. Other schools are currently experimenting with a three-year program for select students.

In Their Own Words: What Medical School Admissions Officers Say

During the four years I'd spent at Wake Forest University School of Medicine, and over the years since, I've had the opportunity to speak with many medical school faculty members and admissions officers. The following are some or their thoughts about the admissions process, what schools are specifically looking for in applicants, and what the trends are for the future. The answers are a compilation of the most common responses.

Q. How are the admissions criteria today different than they were 5 or 10 years ago?

A. We're looking more at the whole individual and not just looking at numbers. Of course we want students who are intelligent and motivated, and who demonstrate that by having good grades, but we also want individuals who are well-rounded and will add something to the class. Ten or twenty years ago, I don't think we thought much about personality or social skills, but now we do. The interview process looks more deeply into an applicant's ability to connect with people.

Q. What are you specifically looking for in today's medical school applicant?

A. We want critical thinkers, problem solvers, and team players. You can't diagnose diseases or solve today's medical issues unless you think critically. You also need to be a team player because that's where medical education and medicine is heading. Being a loner is out; being part of a team that gets things done is in.

Q. What are the top 3 qualities you're looking for in an applicant?

A. Intelligence, a great work ethic, and empathy. Let's face it; medicine is science. And unless you're good at science, you're not going to make it through medical school. That's why GPA and MCAT scores are so important –they're a gauge of how well a student will do during the first year of medical school. To get through medical school requires sacrifice, long hours, and a great work ethic. Unless you work really hard, you're not going to make it. You also need empathy for others. No matter how good you are at medicine, being a good doctor means you also have to be an empathetic and compassionate human being.

Q. Why are most applicants rejected?

A. No matter how much we like an applicant, and believe he or she has the personality to be a good doctor, the bottom line is grades. If a student can't do well in college, how are they ever going to get through medical school? Sometimes we look at trends and see if a student has improved from his or her freshman year, and what circumstances could have prevented the student from doing well early on. But grades become increasingly important as a student progresses through college. We can forgive a poor start, but we don't look favorably on continued poor performance. In the end, a student's overall and science GPA are more important than freshman performance.

Q. Why is the MCAT so important?

A. There's a lot of competition for slots in medical school, and we want to make sure that we graduate the highest number of students we can. The MCAT is one of the best ways to predict how much difficulty a student will have getting through medical school and how well they will do on their licensure exams. Another important factor is how the MCAT scores compare with the academic record. If there's a significant difference, it raises questions. High MCAT scores and poor grades may indicate good potential but laziness. Low MCAT scores may indicate that the student tests well in class but may not have the critical thinking skills needed for a medical curriculum.

Q. What are the things that students should really focus on to become top candidates?

A. Nothing guarantees a student will get admitted to medical school. There are students with 3.8 GPAs that don't get in and there are students with 3.0 GPAs that do. Naturally, the chances are much better if grades are high, but admissions committees look at personal qualities, maturity, life experience, motivation, and challenges that a student had to face while in school. It's important for students to demonstrate their interest in medicine by volunteering and doing community service, especially in health-related activities. So, I would focus on becoming a well-rounded applicant who shows leadership skills, an ability to work with others, and someone who's committed to becoming a physician. That said, a student should not neglect his or her grades, since academic performance is really the true test of how well that student can handle a medical curriculum.

Top Five Reasons Applicants are Rejected

Every year, thousands of medical school applicants are rejected for a variety of reasons. We've already covered the most important criteria medical schools look for, but according to medical school admissions officers there are five main reasons why medical schools will reject an applicant. They are:

1. **Poor grades and/or MCAT scores.** Many schools screen applicants based on minimum GPA and MCAT scores and will automatically reject an applicant that falls below a certain threshold. The general rule of thumb is that you should have an overall GPA of 3.5 with a strong performance in the sciences and a minimum overall score above 500 on the MCAT. If your MCAT scores are lower (not much lower) but your GPA is outstanding, especially if your undergraduate school was rigorous and competitive, your chances are better.
2. **Lack of clinical experience.** One of the common questions an admissions committee member will ask is, "How can this applicant possibly know that he or she wants to be a doctor if he or she has never spent a reasonable amount of time in a clinical setting?" If you're applying to medical school, you better demonstrate your interest through clinical experiences. It's difficult to convince someone looking at your application or interviewing you that you're serious about medicine if you have not done anything to prove it. The most favorable applicants have shadowed doctors, volunteered at clinics or hospitals, or participated in premed programs that included time spent with physicians.
3. **Narrow choice of schools.** Unless a student has outstanding grades, remarkably high MCAT scores, exceptional extracurricular activities, and excellent interview skills, he or she must apply to a wide range of medical schools. Competition is fierce. Some national schools receive more than 14,000 applications and are very selective in who they accept. You may think that a 3.5 GPA and a score of 510 on the MCAT will get you into Harvard or Duke, but it most likely will not. So cover all your bases and include both your dream medical schools and five to seven less selective schools that would more likely accept you, given your academic record.
4. **Poorly written essay.** Sometimes the difference between getting an interview and an outright rejection comes down to the essay. In borderline cases, an essay will certainly convince an admissions committee member that you're someone who deserves further consideration. A poorly written essay, on the other hand, will make

the rest of your application seem less desirable. If it doesn't answer the questions of why you want to be a doctor, what led you to this decision, and what you've done to cultivate your interest in medicine, your application will simply be one of the thousands that are rejected.

5. **Poor interview skills.** The last step in the process is the medical school interview, which can be a make or break event for some applicants. This is the last chance an admissions committee member has to get to know the applicant and answer any questions or any lingering doubts about academics, volunteer work, desire to be a doctor, etc. It's also an opportunity for the applicant to make a convincing argument as to why he or she would make a good candidate for the school's program. Getting this far into the process is a good sign, but some applicants who would otherwise get accepted fall short simply because they're not prepared or didn't practice beforehand. Don't assume that the interview is simply a formality. Take it seriously.

Schools with the Best Chances for Successful Admission

The number of U.S. medical schools has increased to 155, with several more under consideration or ready to begin enrolling students over the next few years. According to the experts, by 2025 first-year medical school enrollment is projected to reach 23,000, an increase of 30 percent from 2002. This doesn't mean medical schools are lowering their standards, since the number of applicants is also increasing accordingly. Students must still apply wisely and select schools that will give them the best chance for admission.

By far, your best chance of being accepted is with a medical school in your own state of residence. On average, state medical schools accept about 90 percent state residents and, therefore, will accept only a few, "very well qualified" non-resident applicants. Even some of the privately-owned medical schools that receive financial assistance from the state in which they're located are expected to accept a good percentage of state residents.

What it comes down to is that medical schools usually have two unofficial applicant pools: an in-state applicant pool and an out-of-state applicant pool. Because of higher admissions criteria, out-of-state applicants generally have higher GPAs and MCAT scores and, therefore, in-state applicants would not do as well if they were compared with the usually more competitive out-of-state applicant pool. This doesn't mean that you should not apply to any medical school you'd like, but you should realize that the odds are much more in your favor with schools in your own state of residence.

If you're well qualified (above average grades, high MCAT scores, excellent letters of evaluation, and a good record of extracurricular activities), then you may very well be a candidate for one of the "national" schools such as Harvard, Duke, Johns Hopkins, etc. If your credentials are not superior, however, your best bet is to look at schools in your own state and also at some of the less prestigious schools around the country, which don't receive as many applications but that are trying to attract good quality students.

Remember, the larger the applicant pool, the less your chances become unless you're an outstanding candidate. Some of the well-known medical schools receiving thousands of applications a year can certainly be more selective than a school that receives only 800. The former will almost always draw the line at grades and MCAT scores to cut the field down. So, if your grades and MCAT scores are not superior, your chances of getting very far in the selection process are slim to none.

If your primary goal is to become a doctor, but your qualifications are not the best, don't be concerned about which medical school you'll be going to. Instead, concentrate your efforts on getting into a medical school period. Obtain a copy of the Medical School Admission Requirements from the AAMC, as well as literature from individual medical schools. Examine your choices realistically based on your qualifications and the medical school's selection criteria. Talk to your premedical advisor about your chances of getting into a particular medical school and save yourself a lot of time and effort by choosing medical schools carefully and sensibly.

There's no doubt that many good students are not physicians today because they were either too narrow-minded about which school they wanted to attend, or they didn't see their realistic chances of being accepted to certain medical schools. Let's face it; the student who seriously considers a career in medicine shouldn't be too concerned about the school's name on the diploma. How many times have you asked your doctor the name of the medical school he or she attended? When you begin practicing medicine, or unless your goal is to work at a prestigious national medical center, the name of the medical school you graduated from will be insignificant.

In summary, when it comes down to which schools you should apply to, there are three basic strategies that are effective in boosting your overall probability for acceptance:

- Unless you're in the top 10-20 percent of all students nationwide, you should always give first consideration to your state-of-residence medical schools. Oddly enough, students with less than stellar credentials still apply to medical schools that accept less than five percent non-residents! Even someone in the top 10 percent is probably not getting into those schools. Examine the ratios of resident to non-resident acceptance rates at various medical schools and apply accordingly.
- Be realistic when it comes to applying to nationally prestigious medical schools. I suspect most students would like to attend Harvard, Yale, or Johns Hopkins. Realistically, very few have the credentials to even get through the initial screening process. Look carefully at your GPA, MCAT scores, background, and the competitiveness of your undergraduate institution. All things being equal, your undergraduate school is a key factor in how medical schools view the rest of your qualifications. The more competitive the undergraduate program, the better your chances become.
- Always consider the stated mission of the medical school and how that mission fits in with your application profile. For example, a medical school's principle mission may be to train general practitioners for the state and would like applicants who have had experience in the health care field. Even though you may have a good GPA and are a

state resident, you may not "fit" the mission of the school or you may not be suited to their program because you lack certain background qualifications. Before applying, review that school's brochure or catalogue and make sure your profile matches the aims and goals of that school. This can save you a lot of time and energy.

Examples of Medical School Admission Rates

The issue of acceptance rates can sometimes be misleading, and it can cause a student to not apply to a particular school. First, don't be intimidated when you hear that medical school is so difficult to get into that only a small percentage of applicants are successful. The truth is that each year more than 40 percent of applicants are accepted; and unless you have a poor academic record and no extracurricular activities to demonstrate that you're serious about a career in medicine, your chances of getting admitted somewhere are fairly good. The problem often lies in where you apply. If you're a resident of one state and you apply to a school in another state that accepts 98 percent residents, your chances are near zero.

In order to help you get an idea of which medical schools over the past few years have had the best acceptance records for residents, non-residents, and women students, I've included the following tables based on recent statistics compiled by the AAMC and other sources. Use these only as a guide in helping make school selections, since admissions criteria change year to year and from committee to committee. Some medical schools have such a reputation for being selective that many applicants don't even waste their time and money applying. On the other hand, some less selective schools attract more applicants because they're more open to considering students outside their state.

The latest edition of the AAMC's Medical School Admission Requirements will have the very latest statistics. However, never feel that you shouldn't apply to a particular school based only on numbers. Apply to any medical school you'd like, but also apply to schools that will give you a little extra insurance in terms of success rate.

Medical Schools with Incoming Classes of more than 75 percent Non-Residents, 2024-25

Medical School	Residents	Non-Residents
Howard University	0.0%	100%
Yale University	1.0%	99.0%
George Washington University	3.0%	97.0%
Dartmouth University – Geisel	4.2%	95.8%
Creighton University	5.2%	94.8%
Vanderbilt University	5.8%	94.2%

Georgetown University	6.4%	93.6%
Washington University – St. Louis	10.5%	89.5%
Uniformed Services University – Herbert	10.7%	89.3%
NYU - Grossman	11.5%	88.5%
Mayo – Alix	12.3%	87.7%
University of Pennsylvania – Perelman	12.3%	87.7%
Johns Hopkins University	12.4%	87.6%
Brown University – Alpert	13.2%	86.8%
University of Chicago – Pritzker	13.2%	86.8%
Duke University	13.4%	86.6%
Harvard University	13.9%	86.1%
Columbia University - Vagelos	14.6%	85.5%
Case Western University	16.7%	83.3%
Rush University	16.7%	83.3%
Tulane University	20.5%	79.5%
Boston University	20.7%	79.3%
University of St. Louis	21.0%	79.0%
Meharry University	21.2%	78.8%
Drexel University	22.8%	77.2%
University of Illinois - Carle	23.4%	76.6%
Cornell University - Weill	24.5%	75.5%

Medical Schools with Incoming Classes of 50 to 75 percent Non-Residents, 2024-25		
Medical School	**Residents**	**Non-Residents**
University of Vermont	25.8%	74.2%
TCU – Burnett	26.7%	73.3%
University of Rochester	27.5%	72.5%

Jefferson – Kimmel	29.2%	70.8%
Virginia Tech – Carillion	29.4%	70.6%
University of Pittsburgh	29.7%	70.3%
Belmont – Frist	30.0%	70.0%
Wake Forest University	33.4%	67.6%
Northwestern University	34.3%	65.7%
Albany Medical College	35.0%	65.0%
Penn State University	35.6%	64.4%
Stanford University	36.7%	63.3%
Loyola University Chicago – Stritch	37.1%	62.9%
Emory University	38.7%	61.3%
University of Michigan	39.2%	60.8%
Temple University	41.6%	58.4%
Western Michigan – Stryker	44.2%	55.8%
Albert Einstein	44.2%	55.8%
New York Medical	46.1%	53,9%
Chicago Medical - Franklin	47.8%	52.2%
Marshall University	47.8%	52.2%
University of Washington	49.5%	50.5%
Medical College of Wisconsin	50.0%	50.0%

Medical Schools with the Highest Percent of Women Matriculants, 2024-25		
Medical School	**% Women Matriculants**	**No. Women Applicants**
University of Texas – Tyler	75.0%	2,070
Washington State University	73.8%	679
University of Massachusetts	71.5%	3,064
Emory University	71.2%	7,046

Duke University	70.3%	4,485
CUNY	69.3%	NA
University of Hawaii	68.8%	1,351
Rutgers University – RW Johnson	67.3%	3,399
Florida State University	66.7%	3,787
University of Texas, Houston - Fertitta	66.7%	2,667
Loyola University - Stritch	66.5%	6,865
University of California – San Diego	66.0%	4,732
University of Missouri – Kansas City	65.4%	944
Quinnipiac – Netter	65.3%	4,254
Penn State University	64.8%	6,168
University of Minnesota	64.8%	3,149
University of California – Davis	64.2%	4,732
Morehouse University	63.6%	4,377
University of Arizona	63.6%	3,804
University of California - Irvine	63.2%	3,874
Georgetown University	62.7%	9,146
Wake Forest University	62.1%	6,443
Oakland Beaumont University	61.6%	4,083
LSU University – New Orleans	61.5%	2,222
Southern Illinois University	61.3%	605
East Carolina University	61.1%	635
SUNY – Upstate	61.1%	717
Tulane University	61.1%	3,210
University of Buffalo- Jacobs	60.9%	3,445
Drew University	60.7%	636
Tufts University	59.9%	8,043
University of Maryland	59.9%	3,200

University of North Carolina – Chapel Hill	59.8%	3,183
Brown University - Alpert	59.7%	4,942
University of Washington	59.7%	3,894
Central Michigan University	59.6%	4,457
University of California – San Francisco	59.5%	4,813
UCLA – Geffen	59.4%	7,303
University of Oregon	59.3%	3,523
Medical University of South Carolina	58.7%	2,079
University of Alabama – Heersink	58.6%	2,384

Medical Schools with the Highest Acceptance Rates of In-State Applications, 2024-25

Medical School	In-State Applicants	In-State Matriculants	Success Rate
University of Arkansas	319	158	49.5%
University of New Mexico	195	91	46.6%
University of Oklahoma	329	151	45.8%
University of South Dakota	126	57	45.2%
University of Nebraska	261	116	44.4%
University of Mississippi	369	162	43.9%
University of Indiana	739	307	41.5%
University of Kansas	444	180	40.5%
University of Iowa - Carver	295	101	34.2%
Marshall – Edwards	160	47	29.4%
Medical University of South Carolina	556	161	28.9%
University of Kentucky	572	163	28.4%
University of West Virginia	193	55	28.4%
University of Hawaii	219	61	27.8%

LSU – New Orleans	669	176	26.3%
University of Louisville	475	120	25.2%

Medical Schools with the Greatest Number of Applicants Compared with Total Number of Matriculants

Medical School	Number of Applicants	Number of Matriculants	In-State Status
George Washington University	16,370	185	2.7%
Drexel University	15,654	303	22.8%
Georgetown University	14,480	203	6.4%
Tufts University	14,248	202	27.7%
Tulane University	13,443	190	20.5%
University of Albany	12,973	140	35.0%
Temple University	12,939	221	41.6%
Emory University	12,880	150	38.7%
Wake Forest University	12,138	145	32.4%
Loyola University – Stritch	12,060	170	37.1%
UCLA – Geffen	11,326	177	61.0%
University of Chicago - Franklin	11,122	203	47.8%
Boston University	10,680	140	20.7%
Jefferson – Kimmel	10,377	271	29.2%
University of Colorado	10,003	182	51.6%
University of Illinois	9,610	297	65.7%
University of California - San Francisco	9,555	174	77.0%
Medical College of Wisconsin	9,454	270	50.0%
University of Michigan	9,338	171	39.2%
University of California – San Diego	9,267	152	77.0%
University of Vermont	9,301	124	25.8%

Wayne State University	9,159	318	55.3%
New York Medical	9,075	219	41.6%
University of Miami	9,003	235	64.7%
Stanford University	8,998	90	36.7%
Albert Einstein University	8,896	165	44.2%
Mount Sinai – Ichan	8,890	119	26.9%
University of Southern California – Keck	8,657	120	83.3%
Dartmouth University	8,505	96	4.2%
Case Western University	8,441	215	16.7%
Howard University	8,331	125	0.0%
Brown University – Alpert	8,315	144	13.2%
Duke University	8,284	119	13.4%
Pittsburgh University	8,259	148	29.7%
Northwestern University	8,138	140	34.3%
Harvard University	7,890	165	13.9%
University of California - Davis	7,791	139	96.4%
Eastern Virginia University	7,649	151	50.5%
Ohio State University	7,633	217	54.8%
Kaiser Permanente - Tyson	7,593	51	52.9%
Michigan State University	7,582	189	88.9%
Central Michigan University	7,529	104	78.8%
Quinnipiac – Netter	7,345	95	11.6%
Cornell – Weill	7,341	106	24.5%
Columbia University	7,291	138	14.5%
University of Wisconsin	7,125	173	72.8%
Oakland Beaumont	7,043	129	55.8%
University of California - Irvine	6,929	114	83.3%
Vanderbilt University	6,873	103	5.8%

Morehouse University	6,855	188	54.8%

Medical Schools with Highest and Lowest Average GPA and Average MCAT Scores			
Highest Matriculant GPA and MCAT Scores, 2024-25			
Medical School	**GPA**	**MCAT**	**Residents**
New York University	3.97	523	46,1%
Mayo – Alix (Minnesota)	3,94	521	12.3%
University of California - Irvine	3.93	516	83.3%
Yale University	3.92	522	1.0%
Johns Hopkins University	3.92	521	12.4%
University of Pennsylvania – Perelman	3.92	521	12.3%
Northwestern University – Feinberg	3.92	520	34.3%
University of South Florida	3.92	518	61.5%
University of Chicago - Pritzker	3.91	521	13.2%
Cornell - Weill	3.91	519	24.5%
Columbia University	3.90	522	14.5%
Harvard University	3.90	521	13.9%
Duke University	3.90	520	13.4%
Stanford University	3.89	518	36.7%
University of Texas - Southwestern	3.89	516	82.0%
Renaissance Stony Brook	3.89	515	27,5%
University of Tennessee	3.89	511	90.9%
University of Washington	3.88	520	49.5%
University of Texas – San Antonio	3.88	518	85.9%
University of Texas - Houston	3.88	512	95.0%
Oakland Beaumont	3.88	510	55.8%
University of California – San Fransisco	3.87	517	77.0%

Hofstra University	3.86	518	64.6%
Lowest Matriculant GPA and MCAT Scores, 2024-25			
Medical School	**GPA**	**MCAT**	**Residents**
Meharry University	3.46	503	21.2%
University of Buffalo - Jacobs	3.58	507	87.8%
University of California - Davis	3.58	509	96.4%
University of Houston - Fertitta	3.59	506	95.0%
NOVA Southeastern	3.60	506	69.4%
University of California - Riverside	3.60	509	100%
Loyola University	3.60	510	37.1%
Eastern Virginia University	3.60	513	50.3%
New York Medical	3.60	515	46.1%
East Carolina University	3.61	506	100%
Howard University	3.61	507	0.0%
California University of Science	3.61	514	97.7%
Rush University	3.62	509	16.7%
Virginia Tech Carillion	3.62	513	29.4%
Wright State University	3.63	509	66.2%
SUNY Upstate	3.64	510	80.8%
Tulane University	3.64	510	20.5%
Washington State University	3.65	510	92.5%
University of Oregon	3.66	509	73.3%
Drexel University	3.66	511	22.8%
University of Chicago - Franklin	3.66	512	47.8%
UNC - Chapel Hill	3.66	512	85.3%
Florida State University	3.68	507	100%
University of Nevada – Reno	3.68	509	66.2%
Western Michigan University	3.69	509	44.2%

CHAPTER 6

MEDICAL COLLEGE ADMISSION TEST (MCAT)

The Medical College Admission Test, also known as the MCAT, is written, administered, and overseen by the Association of American Medical Colleges (AAMC). For many students, it will be the most intense and rigorous exam they've ever taken. It not only tests knowledge of scientific material but also tests an applicant's ability to apply that knowledge, as well as analyze and reason through complex subject matter. Most admissions committees look closely at MCAT scores to determine how well an applicant would do in medical school.

After dropout rates in medical school soared to 50 percent in the 1920's, Dr. F.A. Moss developed the "Scholastic Aptitude Test for Medical Students" that assessed the readiness of students to complete a medical education. By 1946, the national dropout rate fell to 7 percent. Over the next sixty-nine years, the content of the test was refined, modified, and expanded to reflect the rapid changes in medicine and to predict future success more accurately in medical school. Rather than test for visual memory, memory for content, scientific vocabulary, scientific definitions, and premedical education, it evolved to focus more on scientific understanding, problem-solving, and quantitative analysis skills. In 2015, the MCAT underwent the biggest change since its inception because today's healthcare system requires a different type of physician.

With a few exceptions, most U.S. medical schools require that you take the MCAT as a prerequisite for admission. Some schools place more emphasis on the MCAT than others, and a few are notorious for only admitting students with high MCAT scores. Each year, the AAMC publishes the Medical School Admissions Requirements (MSAR), which includes statistics such as average/median GPA and MCAT scores for accepted students. As you look at these, you'll see that the n top schools require the highest GPA's and MCAT scores.

The exam, which is given most months throughout the year, is a standardized computer-based multiple-choice exam designed to assess science knowledge and problem-solving and critical thinking skills; and it's also used to predict future success on medical board exams. In fact, almost half of all medical school admissions officers surveyed said that a low MCAT score is one of the biggest application killers. Counting breaks, the new MCAT typically lasts about seven and half hours. It's longer than the previous exam, but with a greater number of questions, the scores can be more standardized. Since the exam dates change every year, you should check the AAMC website for the latest exam schedules. The 2020 MCAT was shortened to less than 6 hours, with fewer questions due to the COVID pandemic. In 2023-24, more than 85,000 students sat for the 7.5 hour exam.

About the New MCAT

According to the medical school faculty and administrators I've spoken to, one of the best predictors of success in medical school, especially during the first year, is the MCAT. That's why most medical schools place such an emphasis on MCAT scores. So why did the MCAT need to change? At a time when healthcare and the roles of physicians are evolving, the MCAT had to change to adapt to current and future medical training. And as society ages and grows more diverse, it's only natural that the MCAT needed to include a section on psychology, behavior, and sociology. In addition, some students who did well on the MCAT were not able to apply their knowledge once they got to medical school. The new test involves more reasoning, analytical, and critical thinking skills than it does memorization.

The biggest changes in the new MCAT include (1) an increased emphasis on biochemistry, (2) a new section that tests knowledge and aptitude in psychological, multicultural, sociological, and behavioral concepts, and (3) a section on critical analysis and reasoning skills. These changes have been implemented to reflect new ways medical schools are currently training doctors of tomorrow and to better screen potential applicants. Not only has the overall content changed by as much as 50 percent, the test is now longer than previous versions in both time and the number of total questions. The seven major changes to the new MCAT are:

1. The exam is approximately two hours longer than the previous version.
2. There are more questions per section.
3. There's a much greater emphasis on biochemistry.
4. Chemistry and physics topics are more related to biological systems.
5. The writing sample has been eliminated.
6. Natural science and technology topics are not included in the critical analysis and reasoning skills section.
7. A section on psychology, sociology, and behavioral science has been added.

According to the AAMC, the new MCAT is a much better predictor of medical student success in this new era of medicine and a changing healthcare environment. And because it's a longer test than previous MCATs, with many more questions, scores are statistically more reliable. The following is an AAMC summary table of the new sections, the number of items in each section, and the time limits allowed.

Summary of the MCAT Exam	**Number of items**	**Number of minutes**
Biological & Biochemical Foundations of Living Systems This section tests knowledge of biological and biochemical concepts, as well as reasoning, statistical, and problem-solving skills. Topics include growth, reproduction, homeostasis, responding and adapting to environmental changes, and how organ systems accomplish these processes.	59	95 minutes
Chemical and Physical Foundations of Living Systems This section tests knowledge of chemical and physical sciences and aptitude for scientific inquiry, reasoning, and statistics skills. You'll need to demonstrate an understanding of the physical and biochemical functions of tissues, organs, and organ systems, as well as knowledge of the chemical and physical principles that underlie the mechanisms operating in the human body.	59	95 minutes
Psychological, Social, and Biological Foundations of Behavior This section tests knowledge in psychology, sociology, biology, research methods, and statistics as they relate to behavioral and social determinants of health and health outcomes. You'll be tested on knowledge of how psychological, social, and biological factors influence perceptions and reactions to the world, what people think about themselves and others, the cultural and social differences that influence well-being, and the relationships between social stratification, access to resources, and well-being.	59	95 minutes
Critical Analysis and Reasoning Skills This section asks you to analyze information from a range of social sciences and humanities disciplines. Specific knowledge of these disciplines is not required; all the information needed is provided. Areas include ethics and philosophy, cultural studies, and population health.	53	90 minutes

How MCAT Scores are interpreted

Starting with the 2015 MCAT, scores on the four sections are added for a total score ranging from 472 to 528, with 500 as the average. Individual section scores are centered at 125 with ranges from 118 to 132. For example, if a student scored 120, 122, 125, and 123 on the sections, the total score would be 490, which is below the 50th percentile. Scores of 126, 127, 127, and 130 would give the student a 510 total score, which is competitive. There's no penalty for guessing, so never leave an answer blank. At the end of the exam, you'll be asked to choose whether you wish to have the MCAT exam scored or voided. If you don't choose an option, the exam will automatically be scored. If you void the exam, you will not get a refund, but medical schools won't know you took the test.

The writing section was eliminated on the 2015 MCAT because it proved to be the least reliable in predicting medical student success. Another big change is that there are about 117 more questions on the new exam, which means that you'll be sitting in front of a computer for more hours. On the bright side, test-takers will have slightly more time per question than they did on the old exam. Until the class of 2017, students had the option of taking either the new MCAT or the older version, since most medical schools accepted MCAT scores from the last three years.

Since the new MCAT's introduction was introduced in 2015, it will take a few more years to determine how effective it is in predicting medical student success. However, students should strive to score at least 127 on each section and have an overall score of at least 508 to be as competitive as possible. Based on past admissions statistics, students with scores in the center of the scale are more likely to succeed in medical school and pass their licensure exams on the first try. A complete explanation of the new MCAT and how it's scored, as well as sample questions, is available on the AAMC website. The following are tables of percentile ranks based on a cohort of students taking the new MCAT. Use these scores and percentile rankings as a guide when preparing for the new MCAT.

MCAT Total Score	**Percentile Rank**	**Biological / Biochemical Section**	
528	100	**Section Score**	**Percentile Rank**
527	100	132	100
526	100	131	99
525	100	130	97
524	100	129	93
523	100	128	87
522	99	127	77
521	99	126	67
520	98	**125**	**54**

519	98	124	44
518	97	123	32
517	96	122	21
516	95	121	14
515	93	120	7
514	91	119	3
513	89	118	1
512	87	**Chemical / Physical Section**	
511	85	**Section Score**	**Percentile Rank**
510	83	132	100
509	80	131	99
508	77	130	97
507	74	129	93
506	71	128	87
505	68	127	79
504	64	126	67
503	61	**125**	**55**
502	57	124	45
501	54	123	32
500	**51**	122	21
499	47	121	12
498	43	120	7
497	40	119	3
496	37	118	1
495	34	**Psychological/Social/ Biological Section**	
494	31	**Section Score**	**Percentile Rank**
493	28	132	100
492	25	131	98
491	22	130	97
490	20	129	93
489	18	128	86

488	15	127	75
487	13	126	66
486	11	**125**	**55**
485	10	124	43
484	8	123	32
483	7	122	22
482	6	121	12
481	5	120	7
480	4	119	3
479	3	118	1
478	2	**Critical Analysis / Reasoning Section**	
477	1	**Section Score**	**Percentile Rank**
476	1	132	100
475	1	131	99
474	0	130	97
473	0	129	93
472	0	128	87
		127	81
		126	70
		125	**58**
		124	44
		123	33
		122	22
		121	14
		120	8
		119	3
		118	1

The column labeled "Percentile Rank" is the percentage of results for a typical exam year. For example, 87 percent of MCAT total scores were less than 512 across all exams that were given, with 500 as the average score. For the Biological and Biochemical Foundations of Living Systems Section, 77 percent of scores on that section were less than 127, with 125 being the average score for that section.

Best Time to Take the MCAT

First, let me dispel the rumor that there are certain months in which the MCAT is easier, and that students who take the MCAT at those times have a better chance of scoring higher. The truth is that the MCAT is a standardized exam using very sophisticated statistics and, therefore, it's no more or less difficult at different times of the year. In fact, results that are analyzed each year show minimal impact of timing and individual scores. So rather than trying to game the system, concentrate on what works every time, like how much time you spend studying.

So now that we've gotten that misconception out of the way, the question is when's the best time to take the MCAT in general? I tell students that, first and foremost, never take the MCAT if you don't feel prepared and ready. It's too important an exam to take if you've not completed your coursework or studied enough in advance. Taking the exam when you know you still have some work to do is just a bad idea. For example, many of the organic chemistry topics on the MCAT are usually not covered in a year-long organic chemistry course until the latter part of the second semester. Unless you're brilliant and can learn organic chemistry on your own, taking the MCAT before you finish those topics puts you at a disadvantage.

It takes approximately a month after you've taken the MCAT for scores to be released. So, if you take the MCAT in August, medical schools won't receive your scores until September, and you'll miss the early rounds of medical school admission reviews. Taking the exam between April and the middle of July would be ideal, since your scores will get to schools in plenty of time, and you'll still be able to retake the exam without having to reapply to medical school should you decide that your scores were not as good as you'd expected. Some medical schools give acceptance priority to spring MCAT students because their applications and admissions materials are already on file.

September is the latest that the MCAT is offered. If you take the MCAT in September, and you don't do as well as you expected, you'll have to wait until January to retake it. And because very few schools will consider January scores from current applicants, your application will be delayed for another year. Here are some additional registration tips:

- **Register early**. MCAT test centers can be 100 miles away, so the earlier you register for the test the better your chances are of getting your preferred test date and location. Driving 100 miles can be stressful, so don't start off on the wrong foot.
- **Test early if you want to retake the MCAT**. If you're planning to take the MCAT more than once and still want to get your scores to medical schools by August, it's probably a good idea that your first test be no later than April. You'll get your scores by May and can register to take the exam again in plenty of time to make the August medical school admission reviews.
- **Keep your contact information current**. There may be situations due to weather or other emergencies that require rescheduling. In those events, you'll be contacted by email or phone, and it's your responsibility to make sure your contact information is

accurate and current. It's always a good idea to log into the scheduling and registration system to check on and update your information.

- **Recheck your registration information before the test**. Before your scheduled exam, sign into the scheduling and registration system and double check the address of the test center. Give yourself enough time to travel to the center so that you're not rushing and getting stressed out.
- **Check your credit card statement to make sure you're registered**. Before you can take the MCAT, all fees must be paid in full. Your credit card statement will read "ASSN OF AMER MED COLL," so if your transaction didn't go through, make sure that it's taken care of in plenty of time.

Retaking the MCAT

How do you know whether to retake the MCAT? And how many times? First, you should consult with your premedical advisor. He or she has had enough experience with accepted and rejected students to know how different schools react to certain MCAT scores. Normally, scores for individuals won't differ much from one exam to another unless there was a serious deficiency in one of the subjects included on the exam. Only you can judge whether additional preparation will help.

Repeating the MCAT without showing much improvement is not going to be looked at favorably, and it can work against you. So, before deciding to retake the exam, you need to be serious about improving your scores or you must have demonstrated some other outstanding achievement that will enhance your overall application. According to the AAMC, you may take the MCAT as often as you wish, but medical schools may consider evaluating your scores in one of the following ways:

- Evaluate your most recent set of scores.
- Evaluate your highest set of scores.
- Evaluate the average of your MCAT scores.
- Evaluate all scores equally.

One of the reasons students in their junior year do poorly on the spring MCAT and need to retake it is poor preparation. Once these students realize how rigorous the MCAT is, they prepare more diligently and usually do better. I always recommend to students that they spend 3 to 6 months preparing for the test. If you or your advisor decides that your MCAT scores are not competitive enough, then use the first set of scores as a guide to pinpoint areas of weakness. For example, if you did well on everything except the physical sciences section, concentrate your efforts on improving that area. Retake a class or sit in on some lectures. Spend your time wisely by studying the topics that gave you the most trouble. Here are some good reasons for retaking the MCAT:

- Not having the science classes necessary to understand the questions on the exam.
- A wide discrepancy between MCAT scores and GPA.
- A premedical advisor suggesting that scores are too low to be competitive.

- An illness at the time of the exam that affected your ability to concentrate properly.

How to Prepare for the MCAT in General

Most premedical students don't realize how much time they need to spend preparing for the MCAT. By their junior year, they've become good at cramming and memorizing facts and information in order to do well on an exam that tests a specific amount of material. The MCAT is different. It tests significant scientific content knowledge as well your ability to think critically and to apply that knowledge. Studying for the MCAT is not a sprint; it's a marathon. You cannot simply study your class notes for a few weeks and expect to do well. You must begin three to six months before you're scheduled to take the exam and establish a routine in which you set aside a specific time to study five days a week. A survey of successful applicants found that, on average, they'd spent between 300 and 400 hours preparing for the MCAT.

Besides studying the material every day, one of the best things you can do is take regular practice tests. The worst thing to do is to wait until a few weeks before to take these tests, only to find out that you're not as ready as you thought you were. The more tests you take, the more you'll shore up your weaknesses and the more confident you'll be when you see a steady improvement in your scores. When you take practice tests, make sure you simulate real test conditions, with timed breaks and a clock to make sure you're not going over the allotted time. Students who do this feel less stressed when they sit for the actual exam.

There are several important and necessary skills you must have in order to do well on the science and the critical analysis and reasoning skills sections of the MCAT. Applicants are tested on their understanding of scientific concepts, on their ability to reason through problems, and on their ability to interpret data. Many students who don't do well on the MCAT have trouble with applying the knowledge they have to unfamiliar situations. This is where reading scientific literature will come in handy. Here are the main skills you should work on to do well in that area:

Knowledge of Scientific Concepts:

- Understanding the principle concepts in biology, chemistry, and physics.
- Identifying relationships between concepts.

Critical Thinking and Problem Solving:

- Analyzing passages and looking for viewpoints, arguments, and problems.
- Identifying evidence that leads to conclusions.
- Evaluating and dissecting information.
- Evaluating arguments.

Understanding Data and Using Statistical Reasoning:

- Analyzing data and statistics.
- Drawing conclusions based on data.

Understanding Scientific Research:

- Interpreting tables, graphs, charts, and figures.
- Forming and testing a hypothesis and alternate hypothesis.
- Understanding experimental design and the purpose of a research study.
- Understanding the basic components of an experiment.
- Determining cause and effect.

Preparing for the Biological and Biochemical Section

The main change to this section is a significant increase in biochemistry. In fact, according to the AAMC, first year biochemistry accounts for 25% of the questions and introductory biology accounts for 65%. Much of the organic chemistry that was included in the old Biological Section is now in the new Chemical and Physical Foundations of Biological Systems section. On the other hand, a few general chemistry concepts such as concentration within cells, colligative properties, and osmotic properties have been included.

Besides testing your knowledge of biological and biochemical concepts, this section requires you to use your analytical, statistical, and reasoning skills to solve problems unique to living systems. There are approximately 4 sets of freestanding questions and 9-10 passages that include a set of questions. This is where your reasoning and analytical skills come into play. You must be able to understand what you're reading, link different parts of the passage together, and then reason out the answers.

Key Concepts and Terms

CELL STRUCTURE & FUNCTION:

Plasma membrane structure, osmosis, diffusion, active versus passive transport, endocytosis, exocytosis, membrane channels, sodium-potassium pump, membrane potential, receptors, cell signaling pathways, gap junctions, tight junctions, desmosomes, cytoskeleton structure and function, microfilaments, microtubules, cilia, flagella, centrioles, 9+2 arrangement, nucleus, nuclear membrane, nuclear pores, nucleolus, genetic material, organelles, mitochondria structure and function, ATP production, lysosomes, rough versus smooth endoplasmic reticulum, role of ribosomes in protein synthesis, cell cycle, interphase, mitosis, chromosomes, characteristics of prophase, metaphase, anaphase, telophase, and cytokinesis, mitotic structures and mechanisms of chromosome movement, phases of the cell cycle, apoptosis

MOLECULAR BIOLOGY:

DNA structure, function, composition, replication, repair, recombinant DNA techniques, cloning, PCR, protein synthesis, mRNA, tRNA, rRNA, ribosomes, RNA processing, genetic code, transcription, translation, transcriptional and posttranscriptional regulation, eukaryotic cell structure, gene expression, control of gene expression, gene regulation, mechanisms of cancer, oncogenes, tumor suppressor genes, telomeres, centromeres

BIOCHEMISTRY:
Amino acids, amino acid metabolism, peptides, protein structure and function, protein sequencing, enzymes, enzyme mechanisms, coenzymes, enzyme kinetics, substrates, feedback inhibition, competitive and noncompetitive inhibition, activation energy, metabolism, glycolysis, Krebs cycle, electron transport, ATP production, oxidative phosphorylation, lipid structure and function, carbohydrate metabolism, lipid metabolism, membranes, signal transduction, carbohydrate structure and function, nucleotides and nucleic acids, nucleotide metabolism, X-ray crystallography, NMR spectroscopy

MICROBIOLOGY:
Prokaryotic cell structure, characteristics of bacteria, reproduction, growth, antibiotic resistance, anaerobic versus aerobic bacteria, prokaryotic genetics, plasmids, transformation, regulation of gene expression, transcription, translation, virus structure, size, genomic characteristics, replication, life cycle, retroviruses, reverse transcription, transduction, fungi characteristics and life cycle

GENETICS:
Gene, gene pool, locus, allele, genotype versus phenotype, homozygous versus heterozygous, wild type, dominant, recessive, complete dominance, codominance, incomplete dominance, pedigree, probability calculations, meiosis versus mitosis, independent assortment, linkage, crossovers, recombination, X and Y chromosomes, sex linkage, sex determination, mitochondrial inheritance, various types of mutations, inborn errors, mutagens and cancer, Hardy-Weinberg principle, testcross, parental generation, F1 generation, F2 generation, genotypic versus phenotypic ratios

EVOLUTION:
Natural selection, stabilizing selection, directional selection, disruptive selection, group selection, fitness, differential reproduction, evolutionary success, origins of life, species, speciation, polymorphism, adaptation, specialization, genetic drift, bottlenecks, divergent versus convergent evolution, parallel evolution, inbreeding versus outbreeding, relationship between ontogeny and phylogeny, comparative anatomy of vertebrates, notochord, pharyngeal pouches, dorsal nerve cord, characteristics of vertebrate classes, parasitism, commensalism, mutualism, sexual selection, artificial selection

ECOLOGY:
Ecosystem, niche, carrying capacity, biomass, biotic versus abiotic, r versus k strategists, dominance species, keystone species, autotrophs, heterotrophs, primary producer, exponential growth, food web, biodegration, competition, competitive exclusion, population growth, predation, predator-prey interaction, neutralism, amenalism, symbiosis, biomes, rain shadow, ecological succession, climax community, carbon cycle, nitrogen cycle, water cycle, watershed, greenhouse effect, trophic levels

TISSUES, SKIN, AND THE INTEGUMENTARY SYSTEM:

Epithelial tissue, connective tissue, muscle tissue, nervous tissue, the skin and its role in homeostasis, osmoregulation, and thermoregulation, hair, epidermis structure and function, dermis structure and function, subcutaneous layer, sweat glands, sebaceous glands, role in disease prevention

SKELETAL SYSTEM:

Skeletal structure and function, calcium storage, bone types and structure, joints, endoskeleton, exoskeleton, cartilage, ligaments, tendons, osteoblasts, osteoclasts

MUSCULAR SYSTEM:

Skeletal muscle, smooth muscle, cardiac muscle, red versus white muscle fibers, striated versus non-striated muscle, voluntary versus involuntary muscle, functions of muscles in support, mobility, and circulation, shivering thermogenesis, neuromuscular junction, actin and myosin filaments, I band, A band, M line, Z line, H zone, cross bridges, sarcoplasmic reticulum, troponin and tropomyosin, function of calcium in contraction

NERVOUS SYSTEM:

Neuron structure and function, myelin sheath, Schwann cell, Nodes of Ranvier, synapse and synaptic activity, synaptic knob, neurotransmitters, resting potential, action potential, threshold stimulus, all-or-none response, refractory period, nervous system structure, organization, and function, CNS versus PNS, sensory neurons, motor neurons, somatic nerves, sympathetic versus parasympathetic nervous system, cholinergic verses adrenergic fibers, muscarinic receptors, nicotinic receptors, alpha versus beta receptors, reflexes, brain, spinal cord structure and function, meninges, cerebrospinal fluid

SENSORY PHYSIOLOGY:

Chemoreceptors, mechanoreceptors, thermal receptors, proprioceptors, sensory adaptation, olfaction, gustatory, taste buds, ear structure, mechanisms of hearing, eye structure, image processing, rods and cones, color blindness

ENDOCRINE SYSTEM:

Hormone function, major endocrine glands, where they are located, and what hormones they produce, major classes of hormones, hormone mechanisms, steroid versus non-steroid hormone mode of action, hormone transport, target cells, negative and positive feedback, how the endocrine and nervous systems are integrated

BLOOD:

Composition of blood, plasma, erythrocytes, lymphocytes, leukocytes, thrombocytes, erythrocyte production and destruction, anemia, regulation of blood and plasma production, hemoglobin, hematocrit, transport of oxygen and carbon dioxide, oxygen affinity, coagulation, blood clotting, clotting factors, leukopenia, leukocytosis, hemophilia

CIRCULATORY SYSTEM:

Circulatory system structure and function, heart structure and function, pulmonary versus systemic circulation, arterial systems, venous systems, pressure and flow within arterial versus venous systems, one-way valves, capillaries, gas, heat, and solute exchange, systolic and diastolic blood pressure, thermoregulation, mechanism and regulation of heartbeat, cardiac output

RESPIRATORY SYSTEM:
Respiratory system structure and function, mechanism of gas exchange, role in thermoregulation and disease protection, mechanism of breathing, diaphragm, surface tension, surfactant, nerves associated with breathing

LYMPHATIC SYSTEM:
Lymphatic system functions, composition of lymph, lymph nodes, lymphocytes

IMMUNE SYSTEM:
T-lymphocytes, B-lymphocytes, macrophages, neutrophils, mast cells, natural killer cells, antigen and antibody interactions, inflammatory response, immunity, role of bone marrow, spleen, thymus gland, and lymph nodes in immune system function

DIGESTIVE SYSTEM & NUTRITION:
Structures of the digestive system from mouth to rectum, role of saliva, peristalsis, sphincter muscles, storage and breakdown of food, characteristics of gastric juice, digestive enzymes, production, storage, and function of bile, pancreatic enzymes and bicarbonate, absorption of food, structure, functions and mechanisms of villi and the small intestines, structure, functions, and mechanisms of the large intestines, elimination of waste, vitamins, minerals, glucose regulation, detoxification by the liver, nutritional value of carbohydrates, proteins, and lipids

URINARY SYSTEM & EXCRETION:
Structure and function of the kidney, structure and function of the nephron, formation of urine, composition of urine, countercurrent mechanism, juxtaglomerular apparatus, ureters, bladder, urethra, role of the urinary system in homeostatic mechanisms such as blood pressure, acid-base balance, and osmoregulation, kidney stones

REPRODUCTION & DEVELOPMENT:
Structure and functions of the male and female reproductive organs, differences between oogenesis and spermatogenesis, structure and development of sperm, ovulatory and menstrual cycles, birth control, gametogenesis, embryogenesis, fertilization, blastula formation, gastrulation, formation of germ layers and associated organs, neural development, implantation, dizygotic versus monozygotic twins

Preparing for the Chemical and Physical Sciences Section

The chemical and physical sciences section requires not only knowledge of general and organic chemistry and physics concepts but also an ability to solve problems related to the physical and biochemical functions important in medicine education. The amount of physics material has been decreased, and the physics questions are centered more on how physics principles are used to solve problems related to biological systems.

This section is similar to the Biological and Biochemical section in that it also has approximately 4 sets of freestanding questions and 9-10 passages. The major change is that, rather than the physics passages being strictly about physics topics, they are significantly related to biological concepts.

Key Concepts and Terms in General Chemistry

THE PERIODIC TABLE:
Classification of elements, chemical and physical properties of elements, alkali metals, alkaline earth metals, halogens, noble gases, transition elements, metals and nonmetals, oxygen group, valence electrons, ionization energies, electron affinity, electronegativity, size of atoms

ELECTRON STRUCTURE:
Electron structure, electron shells, orbital structure, principle quantum numbers *n, l, m, s*, number of electrons per orbital, Bohr atom, nuclear charge, ground versus excited state, absorption and emission spectra

CHEMICAL BONDS:
Ionic bonds, electrostatic energy, lattice energy, electrostatic force, covalent bonds, sigma and pi bond, hybrid orbital, shapes of molecules, Lewis electron dot formula, resonance structure, formal charge, Lewis acids and bases, partial ionic character, dipole moment

CHEMICAL PHASES:
Ideal gas, ideal gas law ($PV = nRT$), Boyle's law, Charles's law, Dalton's law, Henry's law, Avogadro law, van der Waals equation, absolute temperature, pressure, molar volume, mole fraction, partial pressure, kinetic theory of gases, hydrogen bonding, dipole interactions, London dispersion forces, phase equilibria, freezing point, melting point, boiling point, condensation point, molality, Raoult's law, boiling point elevation, freezing point depression, osmotic pressure, colloids

STOICHIOMETRY:
Molecular weight, molecular formula, empirical formula, moles, Avogadro number, oxidation and reduction, common oxidizing and reducing agents, disproportionate reactions, redox titration, balancing equations, limiting reactants, theoretical yields

CHEMICAL REACTIONS:
Reaction rates, rate law, how concentration and temperatures affect reactions, rate-determining step, activation energy, activation complex, Arrhenius equation, kinetic versus thermodynamic control, enzymes, catalysts, law of mass action, equilibrium constant, Le Chatelier's principle

ACIDS & BASES:
Bronsted-Lowery, ionization, dissociation, calculation of pH, conjugate acids and bases, strong acids and bases, weak acids, and bases, hydrolysis, equilibrium constants, buffers, common buffer systems, titration curves, neutralization

SOLUTIONS:

Anions, cations, hydration, hydronium ion, solubility, molarity, solubility product constant, equilibrium expression, common ion effect, complex ion formation and solubility, solubility and pH

ELECTROCHEMISTRY:

Anode, cathode, electrolysis, Faraday's law, electron flow, oxidation and reduction, voltaic cell, half-reactions, potentials, direction of electron flow

THERMODYNAMICS:

Energy changes, endothermic versus exothermic reactions, enthalpy, entropy, Hess's law, Zeroth law, first law ($\Delta E = q + w$), second law, bond dissociation energy, calorimetry, heap capacity, specific heat capacity, free energy, spontaneous reactions, temperature scales, conduction, convection, radiation, heat of fusion, heat of vaporization, *PV* diagram

Key Concepts and Terms in Organic Chemistry

COVALENT BONDS:

Sigma bond, Pi bond, hybrid orbitals (sp^3, sp^2, sp), valence shells, structural formulas, ion and molecule resonance, multiple bonding, molecular rigidity, isomers, enantiomers, polarization of light, specific rotation, R and S forms, E and Z forms, racemic mixtures

CHEMICAL STRUCTURES:

Absorption spectroscopy in infrared, visible, and ultraviolet regions, π-electron, mass-to-charge ratio, molecular ion peak, equivalent protons, spin-spin splitting

PURIFICATION & SEPARATION:

Extraction, distillation, gas-liquid chromatography, paper chromatography, thin-layer chromatography, recrystallization

HYDROCARBONS:

Alkane nomenclature and properties, combustion reactions, substitution reactions, free radicals, chain reaction, inhibition, ring strain, bicyclic molecules

OXYGEN-CONTAINING COMPOUNDS:

Alcohol nomenclature and properties, reactions of alcohols, aldehyde and ketone nomenclature and properties, reactions of aldehydes and ketones, steric hindrance, carbanions, α, β-unsaturated carbonyl compounds, carboxylic nomenclature and properties, reactions of carboxylic acids, hydrogen bonding, dimerization, resonance stability, acid derivatives nomenclature and properties, important reactions of acid derivatives, relative reactivity, steric and electronic effects of acid derivatives, strain, keto acids and esters description and nomenclature, reactions of keto acids and esters, keto-enol tautomerism

AMINES:

Amine nomenclature, properties, and stereochemistry, important reactions of amines, basicity, stabilization, aromatic amines

BIOMOLECULES:
Carbohydrate nomenclature, classification, and common names, cyclic structures, epimers, anomers, common reactions, amino acid and protein description and classification, absolute configuration, hydrophobic versus hydrophilic, peptide linkage, hydrolysis, 1° and 2° structure, lipid description and structure, steroids, terpenes, triacyl glycerols, fatty acids, phosphorus compounds, important reactions of phosphorus compounds

Key Concepts and Terms in Physics

TRANSLATIONAL MOTION:
Vectors, speed and velocity, acceleration, dimensions, free falling bodies

FORCE, MOTION, & GRAVITY:
Center of mass, Newton's first (inertia), second ($F = ma$), and third law's, weight, law of gravitation ($F = -Gm_1m_2/r^2$), centripetal force ($F = -mv^2/r$), static and kinetic friction, motion, pulley systems, force

EQUILIBRIUM & MOMENTUM:
Force, translational equilibrium ($\sum Fi = 0$), rotational equilibrium ($\sum \tau i = 0$), torques, lever arms, weightlessness, momentum (mv), impulse (Ft), linear momentum, elastic and inelastic collisions

WORK & ENERGY:
Mechanical advantage, power, work and energy theorem, kinetic energy ($KE = mv^2/2$), potential energy ($PE = mgh$; $PE = kx^2/2$; $PE = -GmM/r$), conservation of energy, conservative forces

PERIODIC MOTION & WAVES:
Amplitude, period, frequency, phase, Hooke's law ($F = -kx$), harmonic motion, pendulum motion, periodic motion, transverse and longitudinal waves, wavelength, wave speed, wave addition, standing waves, amplitude and intensity, resonance, beat frequencies, refraction, diffraction

SOUND:
Sound production, speed of sound in liquids, solids, and gases, decibels, attenuation, pitch, Doppler effect, harmonics, ultrasound

FLUIDS & SOLIDS:
Density of fluids and solids, specific gravity, Archimedes' principle, Pascal's law, pressure and depth ($P = \rho gh$), viscosity, continuity equation, turbulence, surface tension, Bernoulli's equation, elastic properties, elastic limit, thermal expansion, shear, compression

ELECTROSTATICS & ELECTROMAGNETISM:
Charge, charge conservation, conductors, insulators, Coulomb's law ($F = kq_1q_2/r^2$), electric field, potential difference, absolute potential, equipotential lines, electric dipole,

electrostatic induction, Gauss's law, magnetic field, properties of electromagnetic radiation, electromagnetic spectrum (radio, infrared, UV, X-rays)

CIRCUITS & CIRCUIT ELEMENTS:
Current ($I = \Delta Q/\Delta t$), Ohm's law ($I = V/R$), battery, voltage, electromotive force, terminal potential, resistance, resistors, resistivity ($\rho=RA/L$), capacitance, capacitors in series and in parallel, capacitor discharge, dielectrics, conductivity, power in circuits ($P = VI$; $P = I^2/R$), alternating currents, reactive circuits

LIGHT & OPTICS:
Electromagnetic radiation, interference, diffraction, thin films, X-ray diffraction, polarization, Doppler effect, visual light spectrum, reflection, refraction, Snell's law ($n_1 sin\theta_1 = n_2 sin\theta_2$), dispersion, internal reflection, spherical mirrors, real and virtual images, converging and diverging lenses, focal length, lens strength, diopters, lens aberration, ray tracing, optical instruments

ATOMIC STRUCTURE:
Bohr model, atomic energy levels, atomic number, atomic weight, neutrons, protons, isotopes, nuclear force, radioactive decay, half-life, exponential decay, nature if fission, nature of fusion, mass deficit, binding energy

Preparing for the Psychological, Social, and Behavioral Section

This new section was designed to assess an applicant's knowledge and use of concepts in psychology, sociology, biology of behavior, research methodology, and statistics as they relate to these topics. After looking at the characteristics of incoming medical students over the past few decades, experts concluded that one of the qualities missing was an understanding of socio-cultural determinants of health. In other words, students didn't know much about how social and psychological factors influence perceptions and reactions to the world, and how culture and society influence well-being.

The new MCAT addresses those shortcomings and is the reason that many schools have altered their premedical curricula to include these topics. This section does more than test your knowledge of memorized information; it's designed to test (1) your ability to reason and problem solve, (2) your ability to understand design and execution of research, and (3) your statistical reasoning skills. There are five main areas and specific content on which questions are based. These are:

Concept A: Biological, psychological, and socio-cultural factors that influence how individuals perceive, think about, and react to the world.
What to know: Detection and perception of sensory information such as hearing and vision, cognition, consciousness, memory, experiences, how we handle stress, the use of language to communicate, and how we process emotions.

Concept B: Biological, psychological, and socio-cultural factors that influence human behavior.

What to know: Psychological and biological factors that affect human behavior, social and cultural factors that affect behavior, how learning affects behavior, how attitudes and perceptions affect behavioral changes, personality, psychological disorders, learning, attitudes, biology of behavior (genetics, nervous and endocrine systems, how environment affects behavior, human development).

Concept C: Psychological, socio-cultural, and biological factors that influence how we think about ourselves and other individuals.
What to know: Social interaction and behavior, origins of prejudice and bias, discrimination, stereotypes, attitudes, perceptions and beliefs that affect interactions with others in society, actions that affect social interactions, the notion of self and identity.

Concept D: Cultural and social differences that affect health and well-being.
What to know: The relationship between social structures and how individuals in a society interact with one another, social institutions, factors and demographic characteristics that define culture and a society.

Concept E: Social structure and how access to resources influence health and well-being.
What to know: Understanding of social classes, social stratification, mobility, health disparities, and how poverty affects human interactions and availability of resources.

Preparing for the Critical Analysis and Reasoning Skills Section

The fourth section of the MCAT has replaced the Verbal Reasoning section and tests your ability to analyze and evaluate information from a wide range of humanities, ethics, philosophy, and social science topics. It doesn't require specific knowledge of these disciplines, but it does require that you be able to use critical thinking and statistical reasoning skills to interpret passages. To do well on this section, you need to (1) understand what you're reading, (2) link different parts of the passage in order to increase comprehension, and (3) use reasoning skills to apply what you know to what's being presented in the passage. Sometimes that involves knowledge of basic math. Calculus is not required, but the general math concepts you need to know are:

- Basic statistics such as mean, probability, standard deviation, data trends, and relationships.
- Metric system and the conversion of metric units to standard units.
- Analyzing diagrams, tables, graphs, charts, figures, and slope.
- Percentages, ratios, proportions, and square root estimates.
- Logarithms and scientific notation.
- Basic trigonometry functions such as sine, cosine, and tangent
- Vector addition and subtraction.

Critical thinking is the process of gathering material and then evaluating and analyzing it in a disciplined way. Good critical thinkers, rather than simply getting and retaining information, ask lots of questions to understand the material, are open-minded, and use evidence, reason, and honesty to come to reasonable conclusions. To develop good critical thinking skills, students need to go beyond just memorizing; they need to think about what they're memorizing and why they need to memorize the information.

If you're not a critical thinker, you can learn to think critically by asking yourself *why* about whatever you're reading or studying. That's because critical thinking is about questioning; and asking yourself "why" is the simplest form of questioning. Think of it as an exercise you need to do on a regular basis so that it becomes second nature. The more you do it, the more subconscious it becomes. You also need to develop certain character traits. Here are the main characteristics necessary to become a classic critical thinker:

- **Be reasonable.** Don't rely on feelings, hunches, educated guesses, and emotions; demand hard evidence, and then follow that evidence to a reasoned conclusion no matter where it might lead. Get out of the habit of needing quick answers, and instead use facts and reasoned arguments to solve problems.
- **Be skeptical.** By nature, critical thinkers are skeptics. They ask questions, which lead to more questions, and they demand that answers are based on analysis and fact. They also challenge existing facts and beliefs and investigate what they read to come to reasoned conclusions. This will be especially valuable if you're going into a scientific field.
- **Be curious.** Don't depend on a single source for information because this can bias your opinion. It's like watching the same news program or reading the same magazine without getting an opposing viewpoint. If you look at various sources of information, you'll not be as slanted in your thinking and you'll be better prepared to make a decision based on fact rather than prejudice or opinion.
- **Be honest.** Everyone has biases and a point of view. This can get in the way of critical thinking because we tend to ignore what we don't like. Thinking critically requires brutal honesty without assumptions or prejudices.
- **Be open-minded.** Consider all possibilities and viewpoints, regardless of what you might think of them or have heard in the past. This is especially true if a viewpoint is unpopular or has been rejected before. Look for novel explanations, and always be open to alternative or different perspectives.
- **Be disciplined.** Avoid quick decisions. Critical thinkers are accurate, clear, precise, comprehensive, and thoughtful. They never make judgments based on what they feel is correct, and they never look for answers based on self-interest and personal preferences. So don't make snap decisions or go by what your gut tells you.
- **Be inquisitive and reflective.** Critical thinkers are naturally inquisitive because they want to know why as much as what, where, and how. Get in the habit of always asking questions, which lead to future thinking. Once you get into the habit of being inquisitive and reflecting on material, it becomes second nature. To instill curiosity, complete statements such as:

  Some of the real-world applications are . . .

  The key issues involved in this topic are . . .

The main question I have with this topic is . . .
The problem I have with this issue is . . .
Another way to look at this is . . .
What I'm most curious about is . . .
What I find most difficult to understand about this topic is . . .
The reason this can't be right is . . .

Using critical thinking skills is one of the most effective ways to solve problems. That's because you'll have a roadmap that will guide you every step of the way. You can break any problem down and come up with a solution by using the following 4-step approach.

1. **Identify.** The first step in solving any problem is to clearly put it into words and identify what it is that you're trying to solve. Unless you can define the problem and state what your goals are for solving it, the rest of the steps will be difficult, if not impossible.
2. **Analyze.** Once you have identified the problem, learn more about it by researching, reading, and asking others for their perspectives and input. This is the time to drop your biases and be open-minded to fresh ideas and possibilities.
3. **Reflect.** Based on your analysis, consider several possibilities. Now is the time to be imaginative and creative, not closed-minded. Evaluate the effects of each solution, and consider alternatives, even if they seem at odds with current thinking. Sometimes it helps if you talk through the possibilities out loud or brainstorm with others. It also helps to free your mind of the problem and allow your subconscious to process it for a while before thinking about it again.
4. **Decide.** After identifying and analyzing the problem, and considering a number of possible solutions, choose the one you think will work best in solving the problem.

Pros and Cons of MCAT Prep Courses

There are several good MCAT prep courses offered at schools and institutions around the country, but students are always asking whether it's worth the time and the money to take these courses. Based on reviews from advisors, faculty, and medical students, the following are some pros and cons:

Pros

- The online materials are usually the part of the course that students like best. The companies give you so much practice material that you will probably not use all of it. One of the keys to doing well on the MCAT is doing a lot of timed tests.
- You will take lots of practice tests under simulated MCAT conditions and get good feedback.
- The classes keep you on schedule and motivated if you have a difficult time studying on your own. They also force you to prepare before going to the class.
- You will be able to interact with other students in the class, which can help you in reviewing the material.

Cons

- The cost is high, but many students say it's worth the money just for the wealth of online materials alone.
- The in-class study and strategy sessions are not as effective for many students. Those who had taken the prep classes said they gained more by studying by themselves than by going to the class.
- You may get stuck with poor instructors; in which case you'll have spent a lot of money for doing what you could have done on your own. The teachers are usually individuals who have taken the MCAT and did well, and they may not have any teaching experience at all.

Based on numerous comments by students who had taken both the in-class and the optional online portion, it seems that most students found the in-class portion useless, but they highly recommend the online option for the massive amount of materials and the online tests. My recommendation is that unless you're not disciplined or aren't organized enough to study on your own, skip the in-class MCAT prep courses and opt for the online portion for the wealth of materials and the practice exams. These alone, according to most students, are worth the cost. However, keep in mind that all the material in the world is not going to help unless you spend several hours each day studying. That is the real key to success on the MCAT.

Some Final Tips for the MCAT

If you can afford it, and think you really need it, consider the possibility of taking one of the professional MCAT preparatory courses. Even though all the information you'll need for the MCAT is included in your premedical college courses, the critical thinking and analysis required on the new MCAT is unlike anything you may be used to, so you'll have to sharpen your reasoning skills in order to think your way through problems and interpret data. Furthermore, these courses do an especially good job in reviewing the science topics covered on the exam.

Understand that MCAT preparatory courses should be a review of material you have already learned. They should never be your first exposure to the material. If you're going to study on your own, be disciplined. Here are some final tips that will help you get ready for and do well on the exam:

- **Understand the nature of the MCAT**. Don't wait until your junior year to understand the scope of the MCAT and how it's structured. By looking at MCAT resources and knowing the types of materials included on the exam, you'll have a much better appreciation for what to study and how much you will need to prepare.
- **Hold on to your textbooks and notes**. Don't sell back any textbooks you'll need when studying for the MCAT. Also, make sure you hold onto your class notes and other materials that may help you during your preparation.

- **Review course material regularly**. One of the biggest mistakes I see students make is finishing a course and then forgetting about it as if they'll never use the material again. You must remember that the MCAT is a cumulative exam and, therefore, by reviewing material on a regular basis, you'll be much better prepared when you finally do begin studying for the actual exam.
- **Do not wait to begin studying**. Spend at least three, and preferably six, months preparing for the MCAT. If it has been a while since your last chemistry or physics course, it's especially important that you review at length. It's a very difficult exam and one of the main factors that admissions committees use to screen applicants. Find out what works best for you and approach your study so that it's convenient, consistent, and effective.
- **Assess your weaknesses**. Before you begin preparing for the MCAT, take a preliminary practice test. It's free and it takes about 3 hours, but it will give you valuable information about where your strengths and weaknesses are. Free diagnostic tests are available from Kaplan, the Princeton Review, Examkrackers, and from the AAMC. When you take a practice test, choose "simulate actual test" so that you're taking it under timed conditions.
- **Stick to a routine schedule.** When you begin studying for the MCAT, set a schedule and stick to it. I found that students who are organized and set aside a specific time each day to study are much more successful. Here is a schedule from a student who scored exceptionally high on the test. I've added a psychology and sociology review because those topics are now included on the new MCAT.

  Monday: Study biochemistry and biology topics; read two short scientific journal articles and analyze two graphs or tables.

  Tuesday: Work chemistry problems; review physics equations; read two short scientific journal articles and analyze two graphs or tables.

  Wednesday: Review organic chemistry concepts; review physics concepts; read two short scientific journal articles and analyze two graphs or tables.

  Thursday: Review organic chemistry reactions; review biochemistry concepts; read two short scientific journal articles and analyze two graphs or tables.

  Friday: Review psychology and sociology topics; read three short articles in the humanities.

  Saturday: Review your weak areas; once or twice a month, take a practice test to track progress, uncover weaknesses, and get used to the format of the exam.

  Sunday: Take the day off and relax.
- **Limit sessions to no more than two hours**. When you study, never study for more than an hour at a time before taking a ten-minute break. Most students, whether they realize it or not, lose concentration and the ability to absorb information after only one hour of study. Taking a short break periodically will reset your mind and your attitude for another session of studying. After two hours, it's time to quit because retention falls off rapidly.

- **Take regular practice tests.** Use practice tests to gauge your ongoing progress. These tests will identify your weaknesses so that you can concentrate more on those areas. Review and keep track of wrong answers and, more importantly, ask why you got the question wrong. It could have been because you did not know the material or because you simply made a test-taking error. One of the best ways to learn is by studying your mistakes. A month before the exam, your goal should be to do one or more practice tests each week. Make sure you simulate the exact conditions you'll encounter on test day: no music, no friends, and no distractions. Doing this many practice tests will also build your concentration and endurance for the real thing.
- **Use MCAT prep materials rather than textbooks.** Go to any bookstore or to amazon.com and order MCAT prep materials. Use textbooks or course notes as supplements. Test prep companies like Princeton Review spend thousands of hours analyzing MCAT content and are particularly good at presenting only the material that will be needed for the test. Textbooks are just too detailed and contain information that takes up too much of your study time. The only exception is when you need to go back and study concepts you may not have learned, especially in physics and organic chemistry.
- **Use flash cards.** Some of the MCAT involves basic memorization. Going through flash cards several times a week to review formulas and definitions will help. Always keep flash cards with you so that you can pull them out whenever you have some spare time.
- **Do not just memorize.** The writers of the MCAT are more interested in you demonstrating your ability to understand principles and concepts rather than memorizing formulas and facts. As you study for the test, don't just answer the questions; explain them as you would if you were teaching a class. If you know the material well enough to teach it, then you're ready for the test.
- **Study graphs and charts.** The new MCAT is geared toward analyzing and problem-solving, so naturally it includes graphs, charts, and tables that you'll have to interpret. The more of them you're exposed to, the more comfortable you will be at analyzing them.
- **Read short articles in scientific and psychological/behavioral literature.** Because the new MCAT includes a section on the social, psychological, and biological foundations of behavior, don't just focus on scientific articles. Read short papers that discuss social, cultural, psychological, and behavioral issues as they apply to society and its problems.
- **A few weeks before the MCAT, go to bed at a reasonable hour and wake up at the same time as you'll be waking up for the exam**. This conditioning program is important for proper relaxation. It's well known that test anxiety during a long exam is more difficult to cope with when the individual is fatigued. If you must, learn a relaxation technique and use it before the exam.

- **Do not study the night before the exam**. Relax and try not to think about the next day. Get plenty of rest the day before so that you'll wake up refreshed and feeling well rested. On the day of the exam, eat a light breakfast. There are breaks during the MCAT, at which time you can have a snack if you're hungry.
- **Do not eat a heavy lunch**. After the morning session, the last thing you need is to become sluggish for the afternoon sessions.

If your preparation has been ongoing, you'll do much better than if you try to utilize these techniques a few months or even a few weeks before the exam. It's never too late to start, though. Begin now and be very conscientious about your preparation.

CHAPTER 7

EXTRACURRICULAR ACTIVITIES

Because there are more well-qualified applicants than ever seeking entrance into U.S. medical schools, admissions committees need to go beyond grades and MCAT scores to distinguish between good and exceptional candidates. In fact, according to a recent AAMC study, nearly 10 percent of applicants with GPAs above 3.8 and high MCAT scores were rejected by all medical schools to which they had applied. The same study found that nearly twice that many students with GPAs between 3.2 and 3.4 and only average MCAT scores were accepted by at least one medical school. This must have come as a shock to the high achievers who naturally assumed that high grades and MCAT scores guaranteed them admission.

One of the ways that medical schools look beyond good grades and MCAT scores is by considering your commitment to extracurricular activities, especially if they demonstrate leadership, and particularly if they involve work in a healthcare setting. Extracurricular activities can be anything outside your normal course of study, such as full or part-time employment, volunteer work, community service, sports, political involvement, etc.

Any kind of outside activity reveals to an admissions committee something about your character, your interest in people, and your sincere desire to be involved with others. In essence, what you do outside the classroom environment says a lot about you, and it will indicate to the medical school what kind of person you really are. Even if you're normally an introvert, force yourself to get involved, and never underestimate the importance that outside activities will have on your success as a potential candidate. There are many types of activities you can engage in, but the following five are the ones that every medical school expects to see on your application:

1. **Medical-related community service.** This is a make or break activity that every prospective applicant needs. You can choose to volunteer at a hospital or clinic, a blood bank, hospice, or as a counselor working with disabled children, with the elderly, or with the mentally challenged. Whatever you choose will demonstrate altruism and a desire to improve the welfare of others.
2. **Clinical work experience.** Every admission committee wants to see that you've seen the difficult side of medicine, that you know what lies ahead for you, and that you're still interested in pursuing a career as a physician. If you plan to spend the rest of

your life in medicine, you must spend a significant amount of time in a clinical setting to convince admission committee members that you're serious about medicine.

3. **Non-medical community service.** There are things in life other than medicine, and admissions committees want to see that you've spent some time doing something for others and not just for you. When you volunteer at a hospital, a clinic, or a medical service center, you're doing so specifically to enhance your credentials for medical school. But when you volunteer at a homeless shelter or Habitat for Humanity, you're doing selfless public service.
4. **Working with underserved populations.** With the emphasis on health disparities between populations and a focus on primary care, working with underserved populations is a real plus on any application. Many schools are looking for students who will eventually want to practice in underserved areas, so having experience in this area will allow you to discuss on the interview what you've learned and how it has affected your commitment to medicine.
5. **Leadership roles.** When comparing equally qualified applicants, the individual who has volunteered and then took on a leadership position will have an advantage in the admissions process. Some medical schools place a lot of emphasis on leadership, and they require that kind of experience in order to see that applicant as a viable candidate. To become that candidate, you must hold leadership positions in organizations, clubs, mentoring programs, youth programs, or student government.

Non-Academic Activities that Make You Stand Out

In previous chapters, I've discussed the academic side of premedical planning without going into the non-academic side, which can be equally as important if you're serious about becoming a successful applicant. You now know the kinds of extracurricular activities an applicant must be involved in to enhance his or her chances for acceptance. And you also know what medical schools are looking for when examining an applicant's non-academic credentials. Unfortunately, many students rely so heavily on their academics that they fail to realize how important non-academic activities are when applying to medical school.

A friend of mine once told me that her brother was rejected by a state medical school because he did not have enough extracurricular activities on his record. He was your typical bookworm, never becoming involved in anything but schoolwork. So he spent the next year doing volunteer work, reapplied, and eventually got accepted the second time around. When I talk to admission committee members about what they consider important when looking at volunteer work, they all seem to agree on three things:

1. **What kinds of activities was the applicant involved in?** This does make a difference because not all volunteer work is created equal. While one student may volunteer at his uncle's dry-cleaning business, another may be working at a hospital or nursing home. Even non-medical volunteer service such as Habitat for Humanity or a homeless shelter says a lot about an individual because it demonstrates that the

applicant has a heart in addition to a brain. If a student can take on a leadership role, all the better.

2. **How long did the applicant spend on the activity?** Medical schools are not interested in students who spend an hour here and there doing some volunteer work just to get something on their application. A good candidate needs to show commitment, and that means volunteering at least 15 hours a month. It's much better, and more impressive to admissions officers, to pick one or two activities and be committed to them over a long period of time than to pick and choose a lot of one-time activities that don't show much about your dedication or commitment. In other words, be strong in a few areas rather than superficially involved in many. Admissions committees can see right through that.
3. **Where did the activity occur?** In the past decade, a lot of students have been volunteering overseas, which does not give them any special advantage over other applicants, especially if the volunteer work was done in a short period of time while they were on vacation. Applicants may want to save themselves some money by staying home for the summer and volunteering at their community hospital of healthcare clinic.

Don't make the mistake that some students make, which is that scholastic excellence alone will assure you a place in medical school. Start thinking seriously about becoming involved in non-academic activities as soon as possible. When admissions committees look at students with high GPAs (3.5 and higher), they also look closely at their outside interests. What they often find is that many of these students are overly competitive and do not get involved in very much other than studying. When they do get involved, it's not sustained, and it's not sincere.

One of the biggest myths about admissions and volunteer work is that as long as you have some exposure to medicine, especially if a family member is a physician, your chances for admission are good. One of the first questions you'll be asked on an interview is, "How do you know that medicine is for you?" Just because a family member is a physician or that you spent a week working in a clinic doesn't mean that you know anything about medicine or have carefully thought about your future as a physician. The only way to show admissions committee members that you're serious is to have a long-term history of medical experiences. As one medical admissions officer said, "Too much experience in a medical setting is never enough."

After talking to many committee members, I strongly recommend that you devote more time to establishing an ongoing volunteer activity rather than worrying about getting a 3.95 GPA. Until they begin to get rejection letters, premedical students cannot seem to get it into their heads that the difference between a 3.5 and a 4.0 GPA is often insignificant as far as an admissions committee is concerned. What is important is what else you've done while maintaining a 3.5 GPA. The following are some areas of involvement that have proven successful for many of the students I've spoken to and that admissions committee members feel are positive factors in the selection process.

Physician Shadowing

Medical admissions officers will tell you that physician shadowing, although not officially required, is one of the most important experiences a medical school applicant can have. Not only does it teach you about the medical profession and what is involved in practicing medicine, it gives you credibility when discussing why you want to be a physician. After all, how do you convince an admissions committee member that medicine is really what you want to do and that you really know what it's like to be a physician?

Some years ago, I talked to a medical student who admitted that she really was not sure about medical school, but that her shadowing experience convinced her that it was the right decision. Another student I'd spoken to had a different story altogether. He decided, after spending a few months shadowing a doctor, that medicine was not right for him. Instead, he went on to a Ph.D. program in chemistry. In both cases, shadowing a physician was the deciding factor.

Another important reason for clinical exposure is that you'll be questioned about this on your interview. If you have only minimal exposure, how will you explain it? What will you say when the interviewer asks how you could possibly know that you want to be a doctor if you have not had enough real-life experience? On the other hand, relating some experiences you've had with doctors or patients will set you apart from other candidates. Talking about your shadowing by adding some personal stories is a great way to demonstrate your motivation for medicine. Here are some suggestions on how to make your shadowing experience the best it can be:

1. **Find the right physician.** If possible, it's always better if you shadow a physician that you know or have a personal relationship with. If you don't, then call a physician's office, tell the staff that you're a premed student, and ask if any of the doctors allow students to shadow them. If that doesn't work, volunteer at a medical center or a clinic and try to get in some shadowing that way. Many university premed programs and student organizations have contacts with physicians who are more than happy to help future medical students. One of the first things you need to do as a premed student is develop a network by participating in any clubs and organizations that your school has.
2. **Concentrate on primary care.** Because the focus of medicine in the future will be primary care, that is where your main experience should be. Admissions committee members would rather see an applicant shadow a primary care physician (family practice, pediatrics, etc.) than a plastic surgeon or a dermatologist. If you spend time shadowing several physicians in both primary care and in other medical specialties, you'll be indicating to admissions committees that you're not only motivated but that you're making a well-informed decision. During the interview, you'll be able to speak intelligently about your experiences and why you prefer one area of medicine over another. Not many applicants can do that, so you will set yourself apart from other candidates.

3. **Be committed.** Once you've found a physician to shadow, or you've been accepted as a volunteer at a clinic or medical center, be committed to it over the course of months, not days or weeks. Of course, some physicians will only accept you for a week or so, but it's better to have as much experience as you can. In fact, an admission committee member told me that one of his unwritten rules is for an applicant to have at least 30 hours of shadowing. A great way to fulfill that unofficial requirement is to spend your summers lining up shadowing experiences with physicians in primary care and in various specialties.

From the moment you walk through the door to shadow a physician, you must be professional in both dress and demeanor. The last thing you want is for the staff to ask that you come back when you are appropriately dressed. Getting off on the right foot is extremely important because at the end of your experience you may want to ask the physician if he or she would write a letter of recommendation. Letters are important, especially if they come from physicians who know you personally and can vouch for your enthusiasm, maturity, and professionalism.

Athletics

It's difficult to maintain good grades while participating in athletics. This is one reason why you should emphasize this aspect of your college life, especially if you've been involved in varsity sports. Two individuals I knew who were on the wrestling team easily gained admission to medical school mainly because their grades were good and the medical schools to which they had applied knew how difficult the wrestling schedule was. The admissions committee members figured that if these students could maintain 3.5 and higher GPAs in a premed curriculum, they could easily get through the rigors of medical school.

Other sports activities like football, baseball, basketball, swimming, and track, which require students to be away from school and classes during parts of the season are also looked at as good character and team player builders. Again, admissions committees assume that, if these students could maintain high grades despite rigorous travel times and practices, they would certainly be able to handle a medical school schedule. Naturally, other factors are considered before athletics, but athletics can be a positive item on your list of activities.

Academic Clubs and Organizations

Any club or organization you belong to, as long as it's over a long period of time, will make your application look better than not belonging to any organization at all. Admissions committees look at your participation as a sign of involvement with other individuals. A physician is constantly involved with people, and this part of your premedical preparation is seen as a good training period for the interrelationships you will be experiencing during your medical practice.

Debating Team

This activity always looks good on your application because a good physician must also be an effective communicator. If you're a straight A student but you cannot communicate your ideas in a clear and intelligent manner, you might as well forget medical school because you will not do well on the interview. Many upper division classes in medical school require oral reports and presentations before classmates and other faculty members. Even some of the examinations may be given orally. Being on the debating team also demonstrates confidence, poise, and the ability to relate ideas in a coherent and convincing manner. What better quality for a doctor to have than the ability to explain a prognosis or diagnosis to a patient or to a team of medical professionals.

Many physicians are involved in teaching, both on a salaried and volunteer basis. At the medical school I was associated with, numerous seminars were given each day by physicians and students involved in clinical and scientific research. Being able to present the growing amount of scientific information to the public, as well as to the medical sector, is an important part of being a health professional. Showing admissions committee members that you have this quality will improve your standing as a potential medical school candidate.

Science Clubs

Although being a science major is not a prerequisite for medical school, there is still one major fact that many medical school faculties persistently acknowledge: that, in order to be a good doctor, you need to be a good scientist. Medicine is a discipline based on scientific information, observation, analysis, and sometimes experimentation. Because of that, an individual must be able to examine ideas and concepts critically and interpret results according to scientific principles. As a member of a scientific club, you would be demonstrating a desire to actively involve yourself in the field of science. If you participate in any projects or volunteer work, make sure you mention so in your application so that the admissions committee will be able to see your enthusiasm for scientific work.

Alpha Epsilon Delta

Many schools have chapters of AED, which is an honor society for premedical students. Each state has its own chapter, so you can join the organization whether your school is involved or not. The activities associated with membership vary but, in general, the activities include:

- Volunteer work at hospitals, the Red Cross, and other health-related organizations.
- Trips to medical schools to see their facilities and faculty members.
- Seminars and lectures by physicians, medical faculty, and other health professions.
- Resources about medical schools and the medical field.
- Meetings and outings with students and premedical faculty members and advisors.

- Annual convention with workshops, seminars, and opportunities to meet members from across the states.

Non-participation in AED is not something committees' frown upon but, at the same time, membership signals a genuine interest in learning more about medicine. There is a modest annual membership fee, but the price is insignificant compared to the possible impact your involvement in AED could make on an admissions committee, as well as the premedical committee at your college or university. I feel that the greatest advantage of membership is the contact you will make with individuals who can offer help and suggestions.

Student Projects

Many faculty members are involved in various projects and welcome the opportunity to have some volunteer assistance. If you have an area of interest (genetics, biochemistry, physiology, etc.), talk to the faculty members in those departments, find out if they're currently doing any research, and whether or not they're willing to take on a volunteer student. Make sure you tell them that you're offering your services voluntarily since they probably will not have money budgeted for you and will not be interested.

When considering doing projects, do not limit yourself to your major. If a professor teaching one of your non-science classes is working on a project you find interesting, go for it. I knew one premed student who was taking an anthropology course and asked the professor if he could get involved in an urban project that she was working on. It turned out to be one of the best volunteer activities he did in college and helped him write a more interesting and genuine personal statement. So don't ignore what may turn out to be the best experience of your college career just because it doesn't fit the "premed" profile.

Volunteer Work

This area of your credentials is especially important because it shows that you're willing to give of yourself and are demonstrating your willingness to meet the needs of others. Volunteer work can be done in school and/or the community and especially looks good when it involves interaction with people. As a doctor, you'll be dealing with people constantly. Here are some examples of volunteer activities you may want to get involved in and which have been shown to impress medical school admission committee members:

School projects
Tutoring
Student government
Student newspaper
Science clubs
Orchestra / Band
Athletics
Community outreach
Boy / Girl Scouts
Big Brother/Sister Program
CPR / First Aid Instructor
Church activities
Community action groups
Hospital work

A colleague of mine related a story to me about his interview at a mid-western medical school a few years back. The person interviewing him asked if he had any inclination for a certain area or specialty of medicine. My friend immediately replied that he wanted to go into pediatrics because he loved children and enjoyed working with juveniles. The interviewer looked at my friend's records, which showed that he'd been involved in the Big Brother's Program for several years and told him that he would make a fine pediatrician. There was no doubt that my friend's involvement in that program made an impression on the interviewer and was an important factor in his being accepted to 3 out of the 4 medical schools he'd applied to.

Employment

Regardless of the type of job you have had or have now, whether it is full or part-time, seasonal or annual, it's important to include this part of your history on your application. Medical schools expect their students to work hard – harder than they've ever worked before. Anyone who can maintain a good GPA while working will make a good candidate for medical school. It really doesn't matter what kind of work you've done (although health-related work always looks great) as long as you've been a conscientious worker and kept up with your grades.

Often, an admissions committee will examine grades, keeping your employment in mind. If you've worked your way through school, for example, your grades may not be a true reflection of your future potential. Always include any employment experience you've had during high school or college, since this shows that you have at least learned reliance, gained life experience, and possess motivation.

Intangible Selection Factors

Probably the four most important intangible factors medical schools look for when screening applicants are: maturity, leadership, motivation, and sincerity. All these characteristics can be demonstrated by the activities you involve yourself with or the jobs you've held while in school, and are expected in someone who will have an M.D. degree.

Answer the following questions associated with each factor and see how much you need to improve your intangible qualities. If you possess many of these qualities, then you're exactly the kind of person medical schools hope to attract.

Maturity

- Have I demonstrated my maturity by holding a full or part-time job while attending school and maintaining good grades?
- Can I give specific examples of my ability to work with others and my ability to be dependable, conscientious, and responsible?
- Did I accomplish anything of significance (in any field or activity) during my undergraduate years?
- Have I ever shown that I am able to cope with adverse life situations?

- Have I ever had to perform under pressure or work closely with others to meet deadline, etc.?
- If I'm married, am I able to be a successful student and maintain a healthy marriage?
- Do I have to support a family?
- Have I held any positions in school or in the community that require a mature, responsible individual?
- Have I served in the armed forces?

Leadership

- Have I belonged to organizations that served the needs of the community, my school, or my church?
- Have I held any positions of leadership that required my supervision or decision-making?
- Have I ever served in a supervisory capacity at a civilian job or in military service?
- Have I ever been required to analyze problems and make decisions or judgments to solve those problems?
- Have I ever held positions requiring use of communicative skills (presenting oral reports, authoring papers, etc.)?
- Have I been the leader of a group such as the Boy Scouts?
- Have I been an instructor of some kind (CPR, first aid, sports, tutoring, etc.)?

Motivation

- Have I overcome obstacles (physical, financial, emotional) to complete school?
- Can I give examples of my ability to achieve a result because of my self-confidence, stamina, and perseverance?
- Have I taken night classes while working during the day?
- Did I have to work nights after going to school during the day?
- Did I attend summer school?
- Have I worked on research projects in my major field or outside my curriculum?
- Have I done much laboratory volunteer work?
- Can I describe how my interest in medicine developed and how my past life experience will make me a better physician?

Sincerity

- Have I done volunteer work at a hospital, nursing home, the Red Cross, or any other health-related organization?
- Do I belong to any premedical fraternities, clubs, or organizations that show I'm interested in learning more about medicine?
- Have I demonstrated in any way that I chosen a career in medicine to meet the needs of others and am willing to devote my life to helping the sick?

Naturally, many of these qualities can fall under more than one category. The main point is that you need to start thinking about the non-academic part of your education if you're going to be a genuinely good candidate for medical school. If you make a commitment to be the kind of person medical schools want, then you need to get involved right now. Don't wait until your junior year to start volunteering, since admission committee members have the experience to recognize a person who simply tries to pad their resume with extracurricular activities at the last minute just to impress them. I've seen many applicants get tripped up when asked about why they had waited so long before thinking about volunteer work.

Besides, the pleasure you'll receive from contributing your time and your efforts to the service of others will give you a taste of the rewards you'll receive when you finally begin practicing medicine. Hospital work will also give you a true indication of whether you would really like spending the better part of your life around sick people. Admissions committees will see this as an attempt on your part to experience medicine first-hand before making a serious commitment to medical school.

There are two main points worth mentioning: 1) Regardless of your extracurricular record, do not allow your grades to suffer; and 2) be committed in your extracurricular work – don't just do it to get something on your application. Even though grades are sometimes not the final deciding factor, be careful that your GPA does not slip below a 3.2 (3.5 if you're really serious about applying to the nation's top schools). Once your GPA gets too low, no amount of outside activity will get you past that initial screening process at many schools.

If your grades and MCAT scores are good enough to make it through the first round, your extracurricular activities should seal your acceptance. Also, make sure that you don't do what many unsuccessful applicants do – participate in an absurd number of activities that are meant only to fill up their applications. Admissions committees look for dedicated individuals who contribute something to whatever activity they're involved in. Volunteering one day a week for a year or two is much better than volunteering 20 hours a week right before applying to medical school.

Research Experience Makes You Stand Out

One of the best ways to stand out and let admissions committees know you're serious about a career in medicine is to get some research experience. Even medical schools that are not research-oriented will look at your application much more favorably if you have a research background because research indicates three valuable traits that all physicians must possess: curiosity, motivation, and the ability to inquire about how things work. Since most undergraduates do not get involved in research projects, you'll be a step ahead.

At some of the top-tier schools, many applicants are not even considered unless they have some research background, even if they have good grades and MCAT scores. One of the best reasons for getting research experience is that you'll probably get your name on a scientific publication, or will attend a scientific meeting, both of which puts you head and shoulders above many other candidates. So, boost your chances tremendously by starting early. Visit professors that are doing research and ask to volunteer a few hours each week in their labs. It's one of the best things you can do to become a top candidate for medical school.

Extracurricular Survey

The following is a survey I had taken of incoming freshman medical students. I did the survey to find out from the students themselves what they thought helped them most in gaining admission to medical school. Following each question are the answers along with the number of students giving those answers. More than one answer was possible for each student.

Question: What types of extracurricular activities did you participate in while an undergraduate?

Hospital volunteer	76
Community service	64
Alpha Epsilon Delta	56
Physician shadowing	51
Employment	46
Fraternity	42
Social committee	40
Service organization	36
Student government	28
Science clubs	26
Honor society	16
Student newspaper	8
Scuba club	2
Glee club	2

Question: What quality or qualities do you feel contributed the most to your being accepted to medical school?

GPA	96
Motivation	72
Hospital experience	51

High MCAT scores	48
Good interview	40
Recommendations	32
Volunteer work	26
Sincerity	26
Maturity	22
Non-science major	3
Travel	2

Question: What quality or personal attribute do you think will help you most during your first year as a medical student?

Motivation	78
Maturity	75
Proven work ethic	72
Intelligence	53
Desire to succeed	49
Family support	36
Past experiences	25
Other	20

Many of the medical students surveyed participated in or were involved in several extracurricular activities. The common denominator among all these successful students seemed to be their grades and their non-academic credentials, and I would be inclined to say that a student with average grades (3.2 GPA) and decent MCAT scores (508-512) but an outstanding record of non-academic involvement has a better chance of getting into medical school than a student having high grades but nothing else.

The lesson here is that the non-academic side of your overall credentials is equally as important for successful admission and should be taken seriously. Students who are in medical schools today are the ones who learned early on what was expected of them both academically and non-academically and may not necessarily have been any more qualified than some rejected applicants. Don't throw away your future because someone else knows the strategy for success and gets accepted ahead of you. I've known quite a few students who realistically should not have been accepted but who were simply because they knew how to take advantage of every opportunity available to them. So get the competitive edge by being involved in more than just academics. Become that special student every medical school is looking for.

CHAPTER 8

MEDICAL SCHOOL INTERVIEW

If a medical school determines that your initial qualifications make you a good candidate for medical school, it will grant you an interview. All medical schools require an interview as part of the final selection process, so if you're fortunate enough to be awarded an interview, you can be sure that the medical school is interested enough to find out more about you. One of the main reasons for this part of the process is that some applicants may look good on paper but may not be a good fit for the program. The interview is a good way for a medical school to make sure that you're really all you seem to be.

This is also a good opportunity for medical schools to question you about your application, any items on your personal essay, or any discrepancies in your grades or MCAT scores. Admissions committee members really try to screen out what they see as psychological misfits who may not be well suited for life as medical students or as future doctors. Most of all, the interview is a good way for a medical school to see what you're like as a human being and how well you can respond and communicate.

Types of Interviews

Depending on the medical school there are 4 main types of interview:

1. **Panel interview**. Sometimes referred to as the inquisition, this is an interview in which more than one interviewer is present at the same time. The important thing to remember here is to look at the person who is asking the question in the eye and not be intimidated. Because the panel usually consists of faculty from various disciplines, as well as a medical student, you can expect a wide range of different questions.
2. **Blind interview.** This type of interview is given by an interviewer who has not seen your file, including your grades or MCAT scores. All the person knows is that your credentials must have been good enough to have gotten you this far in the process. Because the interviewer doesn't know much about you, expect very general questions such as "Tell me about yourself," or "Why do you want to be a doctor?"
3. **Partial blind interview.** This is like a blind interview except that the interviewer only sees your essay and secondary application but not your grades or MCAT scores.

These types of interviews rely heavily on your background, so prepare for ethical and philosophical questions about your extracurricular activities and experiences.

4. **Open interview.** Usually only one interview and only one interviewer is involved in an open interview. It's up to the interviewer whether he or she wants to look at your file before the interview. If the interviewer has seen your file, expect anything, including questions about your grades, MCAT scores, essays, and background.

Regardless of the type of interview, an interviewer isn't allowed to ask personal questions. If he or she does, you can do one of two things: 1) answer the question if you feel that it's not too personal and you're comfortable doing so, or 2) deflect the question by asking the interviewer why this would be relevant. In either case, don't get flustered if someone asks you something personal. It does not happen often, but it can happen.

Interview Factors

Based on a survey of admissions officers, it was found that many schools regard the interview as one of the more important criteria in judging a potential medical candidate. It was surprising that some of the respondents considered the interview even more important than letters of recommendations from undergraduate schools. In general, the admissions interviewers said they needed to identify the following combination of factors during the interview process. Before going on an interview, candidates should make sure their credentials include them.

- Maturity and motivation for medicine.
- Ability to succeed.
- Interpersonal and communication skills.
- Ability to evaluate medicine as a career in relation to own strengths and weaknesses.
- Academic ability to withstand the rigors of a medical education.
- Common sense or lack thereof.
- Experiences that provide a broad perspective.
- Ability to endure the academic and social stresses of medical school.
- Intellectual curiosity reflecting a love of learning.
- Humanitarianism or concern for others.
- Adaptability and flexibility.

How to Prepare for an Interview

The number one rule of thumb for medical school interviews is to present yourself in an open and honest manner without trying to "psych out" the interviewer. In other words, don't think that you can go on an interview, tell the interviewer exactly what he or she wants to hear, and come out looking like a winner. Every medical school interviews its applicants differently and, therefore, what you might expect at one medical school may be completely opposite of what you'll encounter. Because of the varied nature of medical school interviews, it's to your advantage to telephone the admissions office before your interview and get complete information about the following:

- Is it a panel, blind, partially blind, or open interview?
- What is the normal length of time for the interview?
- What kind of individuals will make up the interview committee?
- Are the interviewers doctors, researchers, or both?
- In what kind of setting will the interview be conducted?

It's helpful to read the school's catalogue beforehand to get an idea of curriculums, teaching methods, programs, activities, affiliations, etc. Knowing the right information about a prospective medical school is important when an interviewer wants to discuss why you applied to that particular school. It's no different than a prospective employer asking you what it is about the company that makes you think you would want to work there. Anticipating questions can also help you prepare by making you feel more comfortable and relaxed. A long list of actual medical school interview questions is included in this chapter.

I recently spoke to an admissions committee member who had just finished interviewing prospective students for several months. I asked him about the kinds of things he looked for when interviewing so many different types of well-qualified applicants. He broke his system down into five areas. Naturally, each interviewer is different and looks for certain qualities when judging applicants. These five areas, however, can give you a good indication of what many admissions committee members believe are important characteristics in medical school applicants.

A. Hands-on experience in a clinical setting: Did the student work in an emergency room, as a candy striper, or with a doctor since all of these contribute to a more realistic understanding of medicine? In other words, was the student exposed to the realities and rigors of medicine before deciding to make a career of it?

B. Knowledge of the profession: Does the student have some knowledge of different specialties and what it really takes to be a physician? Is he or she aware of the profession through some sort of practical experience?

C. Length of time interested in medicine: Is this something the student has been interested in for a long time or just recently? If it has been a long-term goal, what kinds of things were done to accomplish that goal?

D. Personality: Does the student have the ability to communicate? Can he or she talk about relationships? Does he or she have experience in communication either in public or elsewhere?

E. Role Model: Is there someone in the family close to the student who has served as a role model and encouraged medicine as a career? This can be derived from area A.

Interviewing Minority Students

Although the issue of minority status has no place in the interview process, minority students must be aware of problems that could affect their performance on the interview. Unfortunately for the minority student, most medical school interviewers will be non-minority individuals who may have preconceived notions that could be hard to handle. Fortunately, though, there are record numbers of minority students being accepted to medical schools and are doing very well.

If you're a minority student and you encounter an interviewer whose remarks seem to be insulting or insensitive, the last thing you want to do is become angry or confrontational. Becoming angry will adversely affect your interview conduct and make you more ill at ease and overly anxious during the rest of the interview process. Rather than being angry, help the interviewer understand the reasons for any of your past experiences, deficiencies, and activities. Use your background to show your accomplishments and to demonstrate how you were able to overcome difficult life situations and get where you are today. If, after being interviewed, you still feel that you were treated unfairly, don't hesitate to write to the admissions officer and describe in detail your reasons for feeling the way you do.

Interview Questions

The following is a list of actual medical school interview questions I've compiled over the years from faculty members, interviewers, and medical students. The advantage of having so many questions at your disposal is twofold. Firstly, it helps you anticipate the most frequently asked questions so that you can appear confident and poised. Secondly, it will give you a chance to formulate some new opinions and eliminate your weak points as you read through some of the questions.

You'll be surprised at some of the odd questions asked by interviewers, and it's better to be prepared now than to be shocked or surprised at the interview itself. By looking over the questions, you can get an insight into the kinds of things admissions committees feel are important for medical school applicants to at least be thinking about.

Most Commonly Asked Questions

Why do you want to be a doctor?
Why did you choose medicine and not nursing or some other healthcare profession?
Why did you choose this medical school to apply to?
What qualities do you have that would make you a good physician?
What negative qualities do you have that may be a problem to you as a doctor?
Why did you volunteer where you did?
Who are your role models and heroes?
Tell me about yourself.
What about you are you most proud of?
What meaningful experience has shaped you as a potential physician?

Why do you think you are a match for our medical school?
What other medical schools are you applying to?
What are your alternate plans should you not be accepted to medical school?
Outside of medicine, what are you interests and hobbies?
What would you do if you suspected a colleague of abusing drugs?
Have you thought about a specialty after getting an M.D.?
Tell me about the organizations you belong to.
Why do you think your MCAT scores are lower than your grades reflect they should be?
Why are your grades lower than your MCAT scores reflect they should be?
What do you think about the quality of today's health care system?

Frequently Asked Questions

What kinds of people do you like to surround yourself with?
How did you first become interested in becoming a doctor?
What is the most attractive aspect of medicine for you?
How does your family feel about you going to medical school?
How will you support yourself while in medical school?
How will you be successful in medical school and still maintain a healthy family life?
Do you have any idea what a doctor's life is like?
Why should we choose you among all the other applicants?
What do you think is the major problem in today's health care system?
How would you handle a terminally ill patient?
Tell me about your hospital experiences.
Tell me about your work while in college.
Discuss some of the factors that led up to your decision to become a doctor.
Tell me about your family's background.
What do you like about this school in particular?
Tell me about your high school activities.
How does your family feel about your being a doctor?
Tell me about your parents.
What kind of relationship do you have with your parents?
How did your hospital experience relate to your decision to apply to medical school?
Tell me about your brothers and sisters.
Tell me something about your outside reading interests.
What are the negative aspects of being a doctor?
What is your most unique quality?
Do you enjoy being challenged?
How well do you cope with emergency situations?
How do you think your weaknesses will affect you as a medical student?
Do you think your strengths will help you through medical school?
What are some past experiences that you feel will help you as a doctor?
How do you spend your spare time with your family?

Do you think medical school affects family relationships? If so how would you overcome that?

What do you think you can offer this incoming class that other applicants can't?

How much do you keep up with current events?

What do you see wrong with the medical profession?

How do you see yourself?

How do others see you?

Give a brief review of your research.

More Interview Questions

How do you think the health care system will change in the years ahead?

What factors will play a role in molding our decisions on extension of life?

What's the most recent book you've read and what was it about?

Who are your favorite writers?

What kinds of magazines do you read?

Who are your state senators?

How can you be an effective doctor if you admit to having negative qualities?

What kinds of childhood activities did you participate in?

How did you manage going to school and having a family?

Do you and your wife find it difficult during the school year?

How did you feel about Desert Storm?

Why did you select the individuals you did to write letters for you?

What did you do in the military?

What kinds of music do you enjoy listening to?

How do you think society should curb the rising cost of medical care?

What do you think of the admissions process of medical school?

Do you think the admissions process is fair?

Where do you see yourself in 10 to 15 years?

What was your worst course in college?

What's the one question you don't want to be asked on this interview?

How would you affect the health care system?

Do you like to teach?

What kinds of books do you like to read?

What are / were your interests and hobbies?

How would you feel about teaching at a medical college?

What subject did you enjoy most in college? Why?

What is the greatest medical problem facing us today?

Do you think medical school will be fun? Why or why not?

Give two adjectives that best describe you.

Would you be interested in participating in medical associations?

How do handle people who come to you with problems?

Would you be interested in practicing in underprivileged or back country areas?

How would you handle a seductive patient?
How would you handle a drunk patient?
Suppose you had your ideal practice 20 years from now. Describe it.
Did your parents or anyone else push you into medicine?
As a woman, how would you deal with having a family and a medical career?
How would your patients describe you?
Tell me how you feel about medical ethics in today's society?
Why did you go to graduate school instead of medical school?
Do you think you might like to do research as a doctor?
How would you handle a discussion with the family of a dying patient?
How would you deal with a terminally ill patient who refused to take his medicine?
Why do you want to be a doctor instead of a nurse?
What are your feelings about euthanasia?
What do you do for fun?
Trace the development of your interest in medicine, correlating it with your college experiences.
Who influenced your decision about medical school the most?
Explain your summer internships and/or activities.
Tell me about your independent studies.
Why did you choose this geographical area?
Tell me about your research activities.
How can you integrate family life into a medical career?
Do you think high school activities are important in medical school evaluations?
If you had a young patient on dialysis and wanted to discontinue treatment, what would you do?
How did you manage to keep up your grades and be in athletics?
What makes you so certain you can handle medical school?
Why do you think that you would want to see sick people all day?
Does death bother you very much?
Do you feel that a doctor should become hardened to death?
How do you feel about working around patients with contagious diseases?
Do you feel that a doctor should be involved in community affairs?
What kind of social life do you think doctors have?
What kinds of sports are you interested in?
What do you think about public television? The arts?
How would you deal with a patient who refused to pay you?
How would you deal with a regular patient who had poor sanitary habits?
Do you think your extracurricular activities helped you prepare for medical school?
How do you think your major will help you in medicine?
How well do you think you'll do in medical school if you only got Bs in college chemistry?
Why did you attend the college you did?

How much time do you spend studying?
What do you think about computers?
How do you feel about the use of computers in the medical field?
Do you think that computers will become or are already indispensable in medicine?
How would you decide which medical school to attend?
Do you want to get into medicine for prestige and money?
Would you remain a physician if we had socialized medicine? Why or why not?
Do you think that liberal arts courses are important? Why or why not?
Why were your grades lower during your freshman year than during your remaining years?
Would you change any part of your college life if you could?
What kinds of alternate career choices do you have?
Do you like qualitative or quantitative science?
Describe the perfect physician.
How would you react to a patient who insists on another doctor?
Would you tell a patient to get a second opinion if you were sure of your diagnosis?
How do you feel about the rising cost of malpractice insurance?
Is there anything we can do to keep malpractice costs down?
How would you handle a colleague you knew was taking drugs?
How much confidence do you have in yourself?
Would you consider a foreign medical school?
Do you help your wife around the house?
Describe the ideal medical student.
Do you think the best students make the best doctors?
Why is there a drug abuse problem in the medical profession?
Do you know what the divorce rate is among physicians?
How will you handle the stress of being a doctor?
How can the drug and alcohol problem among health professionals be alleviated?
Why do you think people are losing confidence in doctors?
How was it being raised in a large family?
What would you do if you suspected child abuse?
Would you react to child abuse in the same way if the victim was the child of a friend?
Do you think a doctor should ignore his or her feelings when dealing with patients?
Do you think that making life and death decisions makes a doctor callous?
Have modern doctors lost that human touch with their patients?
What do you think patients look for in a physician?
Have you ever been exposed to real life trauma?
Do you think that every student should experience the tragedy of death and disease before deciding on medicine?
Why is your GPA so low?
Don't you think it'll be harder for you to maintain your grades in medical school?

What will you have to do to be successful in medical school?
Do you think that MCAT scores reflect how a person will do in medical school?
Have you thought about serving in the armed forces after medical school?
What was it like traveling around Europe?
What kinds of questions did you expect to be asked before you came here?
Do you think doctors should do much outside reading?
Do you think today's doctors are as compassionate as they used to be? Why or why not?
As technology advances, how will doctors maintain a personal relationship with their patients?
How would you handle a patient who just had a miscarriage and can't have any more children?
How demanding would you be with your nursing staff?
What are your thoughts about the growing number of hospice programs?
Do you think more doctors should become involved in programs like hospice?
Which school activities did you enjoy most? Why?
How much of your college expenses did you pay for yourself?
If you started college over, would you change your major? Why or why not?
Why was your class standing so low?
Would you rather work independently or as part of a team? Why?
What type of person do you enjoy working for?
How many times have you changed your college major? Why did you finally settle on this one?
What courses gave you the most trouble?
Would you be willing to practice medicine wherever you were needed in return for a scholarship?
What do you think about organized religion?
Would you rather watch or participate in sports?
Do you get along well with your boss?
Do you think there should be a minimum GPA for entrance to medical school?
What can this medical school offer you that the others can't?
How can I be of help to you during this interview?
What are your feelings about routine work?
How did you like moving with your family as a child?
Do you feel that living in many places was an advantage? Why or why not?
Which one of your jobs did you enjoy the most? The Least? Why?
Would you change anything about your childhood?
Do you think interviews are important? Why or why not?
What would you do if, during medical school, you decided that medicine was not for you?
Is there anything about medicine that would make you give it up?
What qualities do you look for in your friends?
Give me an example of the perfect job for you.

How much emphasis should we place on your MCAT scores?
What was the hardest year of college for you? Why?
Do you think a science major is important for medical students to have? Why or why not?
How would you handle a patient you suspected was psychosomatic?
Is intellectual fulfillment one of the main reasons you chose medicine?
Do you think the medical profession needs more researchers and less practitioners?
How do you feel about the growing number of specialists?
How would you compare our system of medicine with that of other countries?
Can we learn anything from foreign medical systems?
What do you think the unique qualities of this school are?
Have you read any journal articles lately? Tell me about it.
What have you learned from some of your readings?
How can a physician possibly keep up with all the scientific information available?
Did you enjoy doing research?
Why didn't you pursue a graduate degree?
With all the work you'll have to do, how will you devote any time to your wife and family?
Why on earth do you want to get into this business?
What would you like to get most out of your medical training?
How do think being female will affect you in medical school?
Should dealing with a terminally ill child be any different than dealing with an adult?
Do you really know what's involved in going to medical school?
Do you try to keep up with current events?
Why did you major in English?
Do you think the attitude of the patient is important in the healing process?
How much can a doctor affect a patient's attitude?
Are you the type of person others come to for help?
Tell me about your orchestra experience.
If you changed your major before, why do you think you won't change your mind again?
What factors would alter your decision concerning the extension of life?
Do you think it's in our best interests to extend life?
What are your feelings about performing an abortion on a 13-year-old?
What are your feelings about abortion when the fetus is severely retarded?
Should doctors be willing to be evaluated by their peers? Why or why not?
Why did you work so much during school?
Should we believe your grades or your MCAT scores? Why?
How well do you know the individuals who wrote letters for you?
Do you think letters are a good source of information for admissions committees?
Did any of your military experience help you in deciding on medical school?
Do you think the military made you more mature and better able to know what you want to do?
Are you a self-motivated individual?

How is your relationship with your brothers and sisters?
What do your brothers and sisters do for a living?
What quality is most important for a doctor to have?
Why did you wait so long before going to college?
Do you think that starting college later was an advantage?
With your background, why didn't you apply to vet school?
Why did you participate in the activities you did?
How would I describe the ideal medical practice?
What happened during your third year that affected your grades so much?
Do you think athletics was the cause of your poor grades the first year?
Did you apply to this school because of its name?
Do you consider yourself intelligent or did you have to work hard for your grades?
What have you learned from your research experience?
What have you learned from your hospital experience?
What did you get most out of your extracurricular activities?
Is there one memory of school that stands out more than the rest?
Should personality be an important factor in the admissions process?
Is there a certain personality type that doctors should have?
What type of supervisor would you be?
Are you an introvert or an extrovert? Would that have an impact on you as a doctor?
How would you convince a terminally ill patient to continue treatment if it were very painful?
How would you react to a young patient who wanted to be sterilized?
Give me two reasons why you would not want to be a doctor?
Will you reapply to medical school if you're not accepted?
Would you consider dental school if you're not accepted into medical school?
What's the biggest contribution medicine has made this decade?
How do you think medical advances are affecting the individual patient?
Will there be a time when a doctor is nothing more than a technician?
What will you enjoy most about medical school?
What will you enjoy least about medical school?
Describe yourself twenty years from now.
What kinds of news events have you found interesting lately?
Are you interested in world affairs? Why or why not?
Do you find it difficult studying for long periods of time?
Do you know any doctors personally who may have stimulated your interest in medicine?
What did you get most out of your four years of college?
Is there anything you really disliked about college in general?
What do you dislike about yourself?
Have you been involved in extracurricular activities throughout your entire 4 years of college?

Frequently Discussed Topics

Many questions are asked about things students include in their application essays. Make sure you're well prepared to answer detailed questions concerning anything you include in that part of your application. If you wrote it, then it's fair game, so be honest about your background. Also, be prepared to discuss topics currently in the news. Some frequently discussed topics you should prepare for and feel comfortable talking about include:

- Your hospital or clinical experiences.
- How your family has influenced your life.
- Today's important social issues.
- Current news events.
- Reasons for wanting to become a doctor.
- Modern health care issues such as pros and cons of the current healthcare system, rising health care costs, etc.
- Controversial issues such as abortion, birth control, euthanasia, life extension, etc.
- Discussions about your past experiences.
- Discussions about anything included on your application essay.

I recently spoke to a medical school professor right after he completed an interview with an applicant. He had told me that he gave the student a negative rating based on the student's answer to one simple question. The interviewer wanted to know how long the student had a desire to be a doctor. Apparently, the student's desire was not sincere enough as far as the interviewer was concerned. The student mentioned that one of his fraternity brothers told him that his grades were good enough to get into medical school and that he should try to make it as a doctor. Dumb advice! In the interviewer's opinion, the student did not put much thought into his decision and, therefore, was not sincere in his desire to become a doctor.

Be careful about making dumb comments during the heated stress of an interview. Sometimes the pressure will make you say things you really don't mean or should not say. The best way to get through any interview successfully is to be honest, be yourself, and try to anticipate as many questions as you can to be prepared. Take advantage of all the help you can get, because just one terrible answer can mean the difference between an acceptance and a rejection.

The same interviewer also told me that the two traits most interviewers look for in applicants are confidence and poise. To ensure a good impression, you must be confident and maintain your composure, even when you don't know the answer to a question or you feel uncomfortable answering it. Often, the confidence you show in yourself when you cannot answer a question will mean more than the confidence you exude when answering a question anyone can answer. So remember to be HEP - Honest, Extroverted, and Poised, regardless of the questions being asked.

What students don't realize is that most interviewers care little about right or wrong answers. What they're really looking for are statements that are well thought out, expressive, and show good communicative skills. An interviewer, for example, won't care what your personal views are on abortion or socialized medicine; what he or she cares about is how you express your own personal opinion, no matter what that opinion is, or whether or not it's totally in opposition to anyone else's.

A friend of mine told me that one of his favorite questions to ask is "Tell me something about your mom." He feels that, since moms are a good subject of conversation, anyone with good communicative skills and good thought processes should be able to answer that one well. After all, who doesn't have strong opinions, one way or another, about their moms? Here are how two candidates responded to that same question.

Candidate A: "Well, you know; she's good old mom. What can I say about my mother except that she's a great person and I love her. Without her, I guess I wouldn't be where I am today."

Candidate B: "My mother has always been a wonderful, caring, and humorous person. I don't think that I would be the person I am today if it weren't for her. While I was growing up, she was always a strict parent and made sure that we did very well in school. But even though she was pretty strict, I remember always laughing at some of the funny remarks she would make to us children. Whenever we were sick or upset about something, her humor always picked us up. Even now, we can count on her to cheer us up. My mom never worked - she was always home with us because she felt that her job was raising her kids. She never regretted that. I guess of all the qualities that describe her, the best one would be her devotion to her family. And her devotion to me and my brothers and sisters is something I'll remember for the rest of my life."

I don't have to tell you which of the answers the interviewer was more impressed with. Quite honestly, he thought the first candidate was a lousy interviewee, whereas the second was great. Even if the first candidate would have made negative remarks about his mother, it would have been better than the short, somewhat thoughtless answer he gave. The lesson here is that you need to say something substantial, even if you have some negative feelings. Of course, you should dampen your negative feelings a little so that you don't sound too cynical or bitter. Most importantly, though, say something that will make the interviewer feel that you're thinking about what you're saying.

Say This and Kiss Your Chances Goodbye

Even though the interview is the final step in the admissions process, and most students who are granted interviews get accepted, there are certain things that will absolutely ruin your chances. Don't be one of those applicants who do everything well only to blow the interview by saying something stupid. Here are seven answers that will turn your otherwise great application into an immediate rejection:

1. **I haven't really thought about being a doctor very much until recently**. The most common question asked on interviews is "Why do you want to be a doctor?" If you

are not prepared with a thoughtful and intelligent answer, you shouldn't be applying to medical school.

2. **I haven't been involved in many activities because all I think about is medicine.** If you think that medical schools want students who only think about medicine, you are as wrong as you can be. Telling an interviewer that all you care about is medicine will end the interview right then and there because no one wants an applicant who is that shallow and one-sided.
3. **Your school is actually my last choice.** Only someone who is arrogant and rude would tell an interviewer that his or her school is at the bottom of the list. If that's how you feel about a certain medical school, keep it to yourself! Admissions committee members want students who are really interested in their program. Be engaged and interested no matter how you feel.
4. **I don't remember saying anything like that on my application.** Most interviewers will ask you about things that you've included in your application. If you can't even remember what you've written, you're going to look bad; or worse, the interviewer may think that someone else completed your application or wrote your essay. Look over your application several times before the interview.
5. **I think our entire healthcare system is broken.** You may think that the healthcare system needs to be improved, but don't be so critical that it makes you sound cynical. Instead, explain how you feel that healthcare can be improved and why, as a new doctor, you can help in making the medical system the best it can be.
6. **I think you're wrong about that.** If an interviewer makes a comment about one of your answers, he or she may be looking for a friendly discussion and not an argument. The last thing you should do is tell the interviewer that he or she is wrong about an issue and then proceed to tell the interviewer why you're right. You won't sound intelligent or clever; you'll just appear pompous and arrogant.
7. **I really don't have anything to ask.** Not having any questions at the end of the interview shows a lack of interest. Prepare several questions to ask so that you appear thoughtful and conscientious. The worst thing to do is to say, "Nope," and leave it at that. Applicants who end an interview in this manner leave a bad last impression.

Other Expectations

Many times, interviewers want to see if candidates are aware of the many expectations imposed on workers in the medical profession. The following list of expectations was taken from an issue of Medical Education and should be read several times before an interview. Knowing these will help you seem more informed about your future medical career. You may even want to use some of these expressions word for word during the interview whenever appropriate.

A doctor should be able to develop an effective relationship with his or her patients by:

- Having cultural, social, and religious sensitivity.
- Taking a long-term supportive role in patient care.
- Being sensitive, sympathetic, and equalitarian.
- Developing effective communication.
- Sharing information and involving patients.
- Coping with close contact and emotional demands.

A doctor should be able to demonstrate technical competence by:

- Keeping up to date with developments in health care.
- Being flexible and receptive to new medical ideas.
- Learning to cope with uncertainty and limitations.
- Understanding the process of decision-making.
- Managing emotional and psychological problems.

A doctor should be able to display professional responsibility by:

- Critical evaluation of his or her own performance.
- Learning to judge and be judged through peer review.
- Accepting the challenge of continuing education.
- Maintaining the highest quality health care.

A doctor should be able to demonstrate social responsibility by:

- Containing the high costs of health care.
- Playing a role in health education and prevention.
- Suggesting equitable and cost-effective health care.

A doctor should be able to demonstrate economic responsibility by:

- Recognizing the economics of clinical decisions.
- Basing management decisions on cost/benefit factors.
- Critically appraising efficiency in health care.
- Using expensive technology wisely.
- Rationing services according to need priority
- Developing moral, technical, and social guidelines for resources.

A doctor should be able to arrange an optimum patient care environment to:

- Ensure accessibility to patients.
- Work as an effective member of the health care team.
- Conduct research to improve health care.

Selling Yourself to the Interviewer

An interview is really your opportunity to sell yourself to the interviewer. According to experts, there are four main ways of selling yourself on an interview. They are: (1) Enthusiasm, (2) Sincerity, (3) Tactfulness, and (4) Courtesy.

Enthusiasm is the interest you take in the interview itself and the positive manner in which you act towards the interviewer when he or she asks questions or discusses issues.

One of the best ways to show enthusiasm is to ask questions yourself. So, before the interview, study the medical school's catalogue carefully and have a few questions prepared before you go.

Sincerity is synonymous with honesty. A trained interviewer can spot dishonesty and phony answers and will give you a negative evaluation because of it. I certainly would. If you don't know the answer to a question, don't make one up; be honest enough to admit that you do not know. I personally think character does matter a great deal, and I place honesty and sincerity high on my list of characteristics.

Tactfulness is important in answering questions that require you to disagree with the interviewer. For the most part, interviewers are agreeable, but there will be some who love to put you on the spot. For example, if you have strong beliefs about the Affordable Care Act or socialized medicine, and the interviewer presses you about why you don't go along with the views of most doctors, don't get belligerent; just begin your answer with a simple, "I can understand why you would feel that way, and I respect your opinion on the matter, but I feel . . ."

Courtesy, or lack of it, can kill the interview before it even gets going. Regardless of the question asked or comments made, be as courteous as possible throughout the interview. Not only will it make the interview more pleasant, it will also leave a lasting impression on the interviewer when he or she is writing down comments right afterwards.

Selling yourself can be easy if you understand what the committee members are looking for and you prepare yourself beforehand. Besides the suggestions already mentioned, here are a few key points that should help you sell yourself and seal the deal:

1. Prepare to discuss your handicaps and weaknesses. Don't be so naive as to think that your records don't show a weakness or two. Nearly everyone has something negative in their background, and your job is to recognize it and be able to discuss it directly and confidently. You may get an interviewer who will spend more time trying to flush out your weaknesses than your strengths. It's more difficult discussing the negatives about yourself. It's also more impressive watching someone talk about their weaknesses with finesse and agility. Always try to turn your weaknesses into strengths, or explain how you can improve or have improved upon those weaknesses.
2. Help the interviewers get at the information you want them to. If you have special skills, experiences, and/or accomplishments that are important but are not being discussed, be on the lookout for openings to highlight some of your best achievements. Don't assume that everyone is a good interviewer and will ask the right questions.
3. Research everything you possibly can about the medical school at which you're being interviewed. Interviewers are impressed by an applicant who has done his or her homework about their institution and is enthusiastic when talking about it. Conversely, they're not very tolerant of applicants who don't know much about the school they have come to for what may be the most important interview of their life. This could be a real blow to your chances. Therefore, know the school, be able to

explain why you're interested in it, be familiar with what the school can offer you, and be able to discuss why you, in particular, would fit into their program.

4. Say only what needs to be said. Always stay on the subject and do not begin rambling about things that are unnecessary just for the sake of talking. You can avoid this by preparing and practicing some of the important frequently asked questions you could encounter during the interview.
5. Always prepare at least 5 questions to ask the interviewer. Normally, an interviewer will ask if you have any questions. Never say no! Ask one or two but have more ready in case some have already been answered during the interview. Asking questions will show interest and is a good way to leave a good impression with the interviewer.
6. Send a thank you note to the interviewer (you should know his or her name) as soon after the interview as possible. This will reinforce the interviewer's recollection of you and will demonstrate that you're interested and that you're courteous. Be brief in your note and don't try to make excuses for a bad interview.

Dressing for Interview Success

Any professional interviewer will tell you that the way you dress for an interview is one of the more important aspects of the interview process, since first impressions are formed even before you open your mouth. Therefore, to start off on the right foot, you need to dress to your advantage. For medical school interviews, this means following a few rules that will ensure you're making a good impression.

Always dress modestly and conservatively. Medical school interviewers are professionals, and they feel most comfortable talking to someone who also appears professional. Besides, what kind of statement would you send if you cared so little about your interview that you could not even dress decently?

A suit and tie are a must for men; a dress or professional pants suit is a must for women. Good colors to wear are blue, gray, black, brown, or dark green. Avoid bright flashy colors, loud ties, baggy or tight clothes, and casual attire. Remember, it's easier for a more liberal interviewer to readily accept a conservative interviewee than it is for a more conservative interviewer to accept someone dressed as if it were an afterthought.

Men and women should not wear cologne or perfume, as this could be distracting, and they must be well groomed. This is not the time to try out fancy hairstyles or assume that just because you think you look good or stylish, the interviewer will think so as well. Women should never have brightly colored nails or wear too much jewelry; men should be clean shaven or have neatly trimmed beards or mustaches. If in doubt, use common sense. Your appearance is the first thing an interviewer will notice about you.

Interview Conduct

Normally, a medical school interview is very informal and relaxed. Some interviewers even like to make it a fun experience. There may be one or more interviewers present, but the atmosphere is usually cordial, and every effort is made to make you feel at ease.

Interviewers are interested in your answers, but they're also interested in the way you handle yourself when asked questions about personal or controversial issues.

Forget about thinking up a "correct" answer, and just relax. The best way to act is to be yourself, since an admissions committee has the experience to see right through any facade and get a bad impression of your character. The following are some things to do and not to do during your interview.

Things to Do

Do make eye contact.
Do smile occasionally.
Do present a calm and self-assured appearance.
Do speak with a firm but gentle voice.
Do arrive early for the interview.
Do exhibit enthusiasm and sincerity.
Do show interest in the interview.
Do be courteous
Do listen carefully to the interviewer's question.
Do be honest if you do not know an answer.
Do be prepared for very general questions.
Do be yourself and always act natural.
Do dress appropriately and conservatively.
Do present a neat and clean appearance.
Do ask a question if there is a pause of silence.
Do thank the interviewer at the conclusion.

Things Not to Do

Do not wring your hands.
Do not sit on the edge of your seat.
Do not fidget in your seat.
Do not put your hands near your face or mouth.
Do not use excessive hand motions.
Do not speak too loudly.
Do not make the interviewer repeat a question.
Do not be afraid to ask for clarification.
Do not worry about thinking for a few seconds before answering a question.
Do not be overly zealous or overbearing.
Do not respond to a serious question with a joke.
Do not correct an interviewer.
Do not look away when giving an answer or asking a question.
Do not criticize former employers, teachers, etc.
Do not use poor grammar
Do not get angry at a question
Do not be passive.

Do not lie!

After the Interview

When the interview is over, you can take a deep breath and congratulate yourself for getting through the final part of the admissions process. All that's left now is to send a letter immediately after each interview and thank the school for the opportunity to interview. As soon as you can after the interview, write down the names of the interviewers, along with some notes about what you had spoken about so that you can thank them personally for their time and to mention how much you enjoyed discussing X,Y, or Z with them. This added personal touch will no doubt make an impression.

It can take several weeks to a few months before you get a final decision from the school, so be patient. If the committees are behind schedule, it may take longer than they had anticipated. Find out from the school what their policy is, and don't be calling the admissions office every week to find out what the status of your application is.

If you've done well on the interview, it will certainly make you stand out from other applicants and will improve a borderline application. After all, you would not be there in the first place unless the medical school thought you had potential. All the admissions committee wanted to do was prove to themselves that you have what it takes to make it through their program and become a good doctor. If you follow the suggestions in this chapter, you will more than likely do better than most applicants and can relax knowing that an acceptance letter is probably on the way.

CHAPTER 9

MINORITY STUDENT ADMISSIONS

The AAMC classifies four racial and ethnic groups as under-represented minorities in medicine: African Americans, Mexican Americans, mainland Puerto Ricans, and Native Americans. The reason that medical schools are actively recruiting students from these groups is that the United States will soon face a significant shortage of physicians from culturally and ethnically diverse backgrounds at a time when the populations in these groups are rising. For minorities, especially those in under-represented groups, this is a great time to consider medicine as a career.

The good news, as far as medical school admissions, is that, compared with years past, there has been a positive trend in the proportion of minority students entering medical programs. Prior to 2000, most admissions committees sat back passively and waited to see what kinds of students would apply. A few schools actively sought minorities in order to increase diversity, but for the most part it was not a priority. Since then, however, there has been a dramatic shift not only in the composition of the applicant pool but also in the way students are recruited to meet the needs and demands of a changing population. Physicians who reflect the diversity of the population are more likely to be more empathetic and culturally sensitive.

Minority Application, Acceptance, and Graduation Trends

During the past decade, the total number of minority students applying to medical schools has been increasing steadily. For example, the number of African Americans applying to medical school in 2020 was 4,430 compared to 3,537 in 2015. For Hispanics and Latinos, the 2020 pool was 3,296. The problem facing medicine is that the pace of increase is not keeping up with the growth of certain ethnic groups, and the percentage of minorities practicing medicine is much less than half their representation in the general population. Currently, there are less than 5 percent Black and Hispanic physicians in the U.S. physician population. For minority students, these numbers represent an excellent opportunity because medical schools realize that under-represented groups bring three main benefits:

1. **Improved access.** Minority students who graduate are more likely to work in underserved areas and treat minority and indigent patients.
2. **Patient satisfaction.** It's well known that minority patients prefer minority physicians because they can relate to them better.
3. **Cultural awareness.** When a medical school class increases minority representation, it creates a climate in which all students become more culturally aware of challenges and differences.

The following table illustrates application and acceptance rates for minority students over a five-year period from 2020 to 2025. African American includes students who also self-identified as Black. Hispanic/Latino includes students who self-identified as Mexican American, Puerto Rican, Cuban, or other Hispanic and Latino ethnic group. To increase these numbers, many new programs have been initiated to help students become more competitive and improve their chances for success.

Applicants	2020-21	2021-22	2022-23	2023-24	2024-25
African American					
Total Applicant Pool	4,430	6,167	4,921	4,672	4767
Accepted Applicants	1,540	2,124	1,855	1,845	1,627
Hispanic / Latino					
Total Applicant Pool	3,296	4,037	3,255	3,177	3,236
Accepted Applicants	1,349	1,574	1,444	1,493	1,357
Native American					
Total Applicant Pool	109	41	52	90	39
Accepted Applicants	39	13	22	36	15
Asian American					
Total Applicant Pool	11,216	13,420	12,719	12,600	13,058
Accepted Applicants	4,786	5,151	5,597	5,901	6,404

Although application trends look positive, there's still a huge lack of under-represented minority applicants at the same time the minority population is increasing at a high rate. Even if current admission and graduation rates for minority students stabilize, the overall percentage of practicing minority physicians will fall as compared to the total minority population. This is especially true for African American males.

The good news is that this is an exciting time for minority students to try and reverse that trend. Medical schools are aware of the potential shortage and are currently seeking good minority representation in their incoming classes. As a minority student interested in medicine, you're in an excellent position to gain admission if you're willing to do everything necessary to become the best qualified person you can be.

Preparing for Medical School

Trends for minority students are promising, but some of the problems these students face remain. If you're a minority student, and you've spent four years at a historically black college, the first hurdle you might face is a bit of culture shock and the anxiety resulting from a loss of familiarity. You might be uncomfortable with a change in speech patterns, gestures, words, and customs acquired by all of us during our social interactions. They are as much a part of our culture as the language we speak or the beliefs we accept and are used when interacting with others in our own culture.

Another source of strain that minority students might face is science preparation. Even though many minority students possess skills and scientific preparation equal to that of any other student, you may not because of reasons that were beyond your control. You need to prepare yourself to work harder on enhancing your science background and understanding. If you have problems with reading, then the amount of reading you'll have to do in medical school will simply overwhelm you.

Remedial courses can improve study skills and are usually helpful in developing better problem-solving and general academic skills. Since many students, including minority students, tend to rely on rote learning, courses designed to help build analytical thought processes and critical thinking are highly recommended. They will also help you do better on the MCAT, which has been specifically designed to measure analytical ability and critical thinking.

One of the most important reasons to improve science preparedness is that, besides having students with outstanding backgrounds, the applicant pool has recently been loaded with many graduate students and individuals from various health fields who now want to go to medical school. As a result, medical schools have a deeper and more competitive applicant pool that is strong in the basic sciences, creating an even wider gap between the two groups of students. To overcome any deficiencies you might have in your science background, or to help you get ready for a medical school curriculum, you should take advantage of any opportunity you can.

Best Colleges for Minority Premed Students

When it comes to supplying minority student applicants to U.S. medical schools, not all colleges are created equal. Some minority students feel more comfortable at one of the historically black colleges or universities (HBCUs), while others prefer a more traditional university. There's really no advantage of one over another when it comes to admission to medical school, as long as you take the required coursework and get good grades and good MCAT scores. However, some schools have excellent premed programs designed to attract the best students and are focused on medical school preparation and admissions.

The following tables list colleges with the best records for supplying minority student applicants94 to medical school, and the HBCUs that supply the most African American applicants to medical school. In the end, however, it's not the school but the individual's academic record that determines admissions.

Institution	African American	Total Applicants
Howard University	116	128
University of Florida	100	872
Xavier University	94	100
University of Maryland – College Park	82	428
Georgia State University	70	142
University of Central Florida	66	382
University of Texas – Austin	64	965
University of South Florida	63	393
University of California – Los Angeles	60	1,199
University of Georgia	56	506
Ohio State University	51	540
University of North Carolina Chapel Hill	50	502
University of Maryland, Baltimore	49	125
Johns Hopkins University	48	494
Cornell University	47	402
Florida State University	47	333
Rutgers University – New Brunswick	46	423
Florida Atlantic University	45	146
University of Miami	44	269
Harvard University	43	243
Spellman College	43	45
University of Michigan – Ann Arbor	43	863
University of Pennsylvania	43	272

University of Minnesota	42	367
Emory University	41	370
Virginia Commonwealth University	41	242
University of Pittsburgh	40	388
University of Virginia	40	476
Florida International University	39	327
Florida A&M University	38	39
Duke University	37	322
Vanderbilt University	37	258

HBCUs Supplying the Most Applicants to Medical School	
College / University	**Number of Applicants**
Howard University, Washington, DC	116
Xavier University of Louisiana, New Orleans, LA	94
Spellman College, Atlanta, GA	43
Florida A&M University, Tallahassee, FL	38
Hampton University, Hampton, VA	36
Oakwood University, Huntsville, AL	31
Morehouse College, Atlanta, GA	21
North Carolina A&T State University, Greensboro, NC	19
Prairie View A&M University, Prairie View, TX	17
North Carolina Central University, Durham, NC	17
Tuskegee University, Tuskegee, AL	17

Medical Minority Application Registry (Med-MAR)

One of the best opportunities to enhance your standing as a potential medical student is to register for the Medical Minority Applicant Registry after you have taken the MCAT. Med-MAR was started as a way to distribute biographical information of prospective minority students such as names, addresses, states of residence, racial/ethnic descriptions, undergraduate colleges, majors, and MCAT scores. To be eligible, you must meet these two criteria:

1. You must be a U.S. citizen or permanent resident visa holder.
2. You must self-identify as a member of a historically under-represented minority in medicine (African American, Hispanic/Latino, Native American, or Native Hawaiian/Pacific Islander) and/or be economically disadvantaged.

Medical schools use the registry (circulated twice a year following each MCAT) as a means of identifying and communicating with candidates. If you register, U.S. medical schools will receive name, sex, age, racial/ethnic self-description, mailing address, state of legal residence, undergraduate college, major, AAMC ID, test date, and MCAT scores. This is a good way for minority students to get on the list of colleges who want to increase its minority applicant pool. There's no cost to the student, so make sure that you register when you're registering for the MCAT. During the registration process, you'll be prompted to either accept or reject the offer to register for Med-MAR.

Summer Health Professions Education Program (SHPEP)

The AAMC and the Robert Wood Johnson Foundation have established the Summer Health Professions Education Program (formerly known as the Summer Medical and Dental Education Program or SMDEP) in order to increase the number of qualified underrepresented minority students preparing to go on to medical school. SHPEP offers students a variety of experiences that helps prepare them for either medical or dental careers. These include academic enrichment, clinical exposures, career development opportunities, and financial planning and health policy seminars. Originally supporting six medical schools, the program has expanded to include 12 campuses. To be eligible, applicants must meet the following criteria:

- Be currently enrolled as a freshman or sophomore in college.
- Have a minimum overall GPA of 2.5.
- Be a U.S. citizen or hold a permanent resident visa.
- Not have previously participated in a SMDEP program.

In addition to these criteria, other factors are also considered. They are:

- Be a member of a racially/ethnically under-represented group in medicine or dentistry.
- Come from an educationally or economically disadvantaged background.
- Have demonstrated interest in serving underserved populations.
- Have a compelling personal statement and strong letters of recommendation.

Each of the twelve SHPEP program sites makes its decisions on a first come, first served basis. Therefore, applying as early as possible will increase your chances of getting accepted. To apply, you must follow 5 steps:

1. **Prepare application materials.** Go to the AAMC website and register for the program. You'll receive an identification number, username, and password.
2. **Request an official transcript from every post-secondary institution you have attended.** The institutions must send your transcript to the SHPEP National Program Office. Their website has specific details about what you need to do.
3. **Request letters of recommendation.** Recommendation forms are provided on the SHPEP website and may be mailed or faxed to the SHPEP National Program Office.
4. **Submit your application.** Once you complete your application, submit it online.
5. **Apply for a SHPEP travel scholarship.** If you are accepted and confirmed to an SHPEP program, you may apply for travel funds.

The 12 program sites across the nation are specifically designed to help students from diverse and disadvantaged backgrounds, particularly those from underrepresented ethnic groups, enhance their credentials and improve their chances of medical school admissions. These programs not only help increase science knowledge, improve study skills, and help prepare for the MCAT, they force students to develop good study habits and teach them how to manage their time effectively. The program sites and descriptions are listed on the SHPEP website, but I have also listed them here.

Columbia University

Location: New York, NY

When to attend: Following freshman or sophomore year of college.

Clinical experience: At least 3 varied clinical experiences for each student on the medical track; Students on the dental track will have a weekly hands-on dental lab.

Howard University

Location: Washington, DC

When to attend: Following freshman or sophomore year of college.

Clinical experience: Four clinical experiences for each participant; experiences will take place at the Howard University Hospital, and Howard University College of Dentistry clinics. There are group clinical correlation presentations and problem-based learning sessions.

Rutgers University

Location: Newark, NJ

When to attend: Following freshman or sophomore year of college.

Clinical experience: Each medical scholar will be assigned a medical/dental faculty mentor and will have at least one shadowing experience in the following specialties: internal medicine, general surgery, OB/GYN, pediatrics, emergency medicine, radiology, and ambulatory care health clinic.

University of Alabama School of Medicine

Location: Birmingham, AL

When to attend: Following freshman or sophomore year of college.

Clinical experience: Students receive a combination of clinical exposure, shadowing, and interprofessional experiences.

University of California Los Angeles

Location: Los Angeles, CA

When to attend: Following freshman or sophomore year of college; priority is given to students attending community college.

Clinical experience: Participation in a community-based health fair; weekly problem-based learning workshops on clinical cases. All students receive practical dental laboratory experience.

University of Florida

Location: Gainesville, FL

When to attend: Following freshman or sophomore year of college.

Clinical experience: Students attend clinical skills laboratories and gene diagnostic labs.

University of Iowa

Location: Iowa City, IA

When to attend: Following freshman or sophomore year of college.

Clinical experience: Students shadow healthcare providers at the university and at local health clinics.

University of Louisville

Location: Louisville, KY

When to attend: Following freshman or sophomore year of college.

Clinical experience: Two clinical experiences for each scholar; clinical options include shadowing/observing health professionals at nearby hospitals and clinics, completing patient scenarios at Standardized Patient Center and Simulation Labs, and participating in clinically related case problem solving.

University of Nebraska

Location: Omaha, NE

When to attend: Following freshman or sophomore year of college.

Clinical experience: Pre-medicine: Clinical experiences include opportunities in specialty areas such as: general internal medicine, family medicine, internal medicine, emergency medicine, pediatrics, and UNMC student-run community health clinics. Pre-medicine scholars will also have a weekly anatomy class. Scholars also participate in small-group activities in the Clinical Skills Center including taking vital signs, documentation requirements, taking histories, and patient/providers communication skills. Pre-dentistry: Scholars will participate in a variety of "hands-on" pre-clinical dental experiences, such as taking impressions and making dental models, participating in an anatomy laboratory demonstration, and working in a dental radiology project. Scholars will also shadow in a dental clinic, spend time in the emergency room, and shadow in a dental operating room.

The University of Texas Health Science Center at Houston

Location: Houston, TX
When to attend: Following freshman or sophomore year of college.
Clinical experience: Scholars will experience clinical exposure through a diverse range of settings like shadowing clinicians, small-group clinical rotations in both the dental and medical settings and full-group seminars with highly experienced and expert clinicians.

University of Washington

Location: Seattle, WA
When to attend: Following freshman or sophomore year of college.
Clinical experience: Physician mentoring; anatomy; Cased Based problem based learning (PBL); suturing, exposure to clinical venues like emergency room, operating room, dental operating room, ISIS (surgical simulation lab) and migrant farm worker camps; lectures on social determinants of health related to healthcare disparities; IULGBTQ health issues.

Western University of Health Sciences

Location: Los Angeles, CA
When to attend: Following freshman or sophomore year of college.
Clinical experience: Students will shadow physicians at Western University Patient Care Center and at local clinics.

The principle behind these programs is to build academic endurance through the "mud on the wall theory." That is, get bombarded with enough information and something must stick. Some programs are designed for students not yet accepted to medical school while others are strictly for students that have been accepted but need extra help to become more competitive.

A typical program consists of very intense 8:00 am to 5:00 pm academic workdays that are designed to simulate a first-year medical curriculum through lectures, movies, teaching aids, supplemental instruction, and seminars on subjects such as anatomy, physiology, biochemistry, etc. Some programs even include MCAT preparation sessions. A stipend is offered, which varies from program to program. You can visit each programs website for information about applications and detailed information about benefits offered such as stipend and room and board.

The instructors at these programs are medical school faculty members, and some may also be admissions committee members. As competitive as medical school is, and as much as they want to attract the best minority students, doing well at these programs will get you noticed and could make a difference in your getting admitted to a medical school.

Pre-Health Summer Enrichment Programs

Many colleges and universities other than those that participate in SHPEP offer summer programs for minority and disadvantaged students. Some of the programs may be more research oriented, but if you cannot get into an SHPEP program, this could be the next best thing to enhance your credentials and add something impressive to your application. The following is a list by state of summer programs (other than SHPEP) offered at various institutions. Always check with your premedical advisor about any new programs or internships being offered.

ALABAMA

Diversity Recruitment and Enrichment for Admission into Medicine (DREAM)

University of Alabama at Birmingham Preparation for Graduate and Medical Education

ARIZONA

University of Arizona, Arizona Applicant Academy

University of Arizona Minority Health Disparities Summer Research Opportunities

ARKANSAS

University of Arkansas Premedical Summer Scholars Program

CALIFORNIA

Health Career Connection Comprehensive Summer Internship Program

Loma Linda University Undergraduate Training Program

Stanford Summer Community College Premedical Program (SSCCPP)

University of California Los Angeles David Geffen Schools of Medicine and Dentistry – UCLA PREP

University of California San Diego Summer Undergraduate Research Fellowship

University of California San Francisco Summer Research Training Program (SRTP)

COLORADO

University of Colorado Health Sciences Center Graduate Experience for Multicultural Students (GEMS)

CONNECTICUT

Yale School of Medicine Summer Undergraduate Research Fellowship (SURF)

UCONN School of Medicine & School of Dental Medicine: Summer Research Fellowship Program

District of Columbia

American Society for Microbiology – ASM Undergraduate Research Fellowship

FLORIDA

Florida International University Research and Summer Enrichment Programs

University of Miami School of Medicine Minority Students Health Careers Program

University of South Florida Prehealth Scholars Program

GEORGIA

Emory University Laney Graduate School Summer Opportunity for Academic Research (LGS-SOAR) Program

Medical College of Georgia Student Educational Enrichment Program (SEEP)

Morehouse College Public Health Leader Fellowship Program (MC-PHLFP)

Morehouse School of Medicine M.D. Summer Program (APEX)

ILLINOIS

Illinois College of Optometry (ICO) Focus on Your Future Summer Program

Northwestern University Feinberg School of Medicine CURE Summer Research Program

Southern Illinois University School of Medicine – Medical/ Dental Education Preparatory Program (MEDPREP)

University of Illinois Graduate College Summer Research Opportunities Program (SROP)

Pritzker School of Medicine Experience in Research (PSOMER)

IOWA

Des Moines University Health Professions Advanced Summer Scholars (PASS)

KANSAS

University of Kansas Medical Center Health Careers Pathways Program (HCPP)

MARYLAND

Johns Hopkins Medicine Summer Internship Program

The National Institute on Drug Abuse Summer Research Training Programs

The National Institutes of Health Undergraduate Scholarship Program (UGSP)

MASSACHUSETTS

American Cancer Society Alvan T. & Viola D. Fuller Research Fellowships

Boston University School of Medicine Summer Undergraduate Research Fellowship (SURF)

Brigham and Women's Hospital/Harvard Medical School Summer Training in Academic Research and Scholarship Program (STARS)

Harvard Medical School Summer Clinical and Translational Research Program (SCTRP)

Harvard Medical School Four Directions Summer Research Program

Harvard Medical School Summer Honors Undergraduate Research Program

Harvard School of Dental Medicine Bridge to Dental School

Health Career Connection Comprehensive Summer Internship Program

Massachusetts General Hospital Summer Research Trainee Program (SRTP)

Massachusetts Institute of Technology Summer Research Program (MSRP)

University of Massachusetts Medical School NIH Summer Research Fellowship Program for Minority Students

University of Massachusetts Medical School Summer Enrichment Program (SEP)

Tufts University Sackler School of Graduate Biomedical Sciences Summer Program

Woods Hole Oceanographic Institution Summer Student Fellowship

MICHIGAN

Biomedical Research for University Students in Health Sciences (BRUSH) program at Michigan State University

Great Lakes Bioenergy Research Program – MSU

Michigan State University College of Veterinary Medicine Enrichment Summer Program

University of Michigan Department of Health Management and Policy Health Management Summer Enrichment Program (SEP)

MINNESOTA

Mayo Graduate School Summer Undergraduate Research Fellowship Program (SURF)

University of Minnesota Life Sciences Summer Undergraduate Research Programs

University of Minnesota School of Medicine Center of American Indian and Minority Health (CAIMH) – Native Americans into Medicine (NAM)

MISSISSIPPI

University of Mississippi Medical Center Medical Cooperative Program (MEDCORP)

MISSOURI

Washington University in St Louis – Division of Biology and Biomedical Sciences Biomedical Research Apprenticeship Program (BiomedRAP)

NEBRASKA

University of Nebraska Medical Center (UNMC) Summer Health Professions

NEW HAMPSHIRE

Dartmouth College MD-PhD Undergraduate Summer (MPUS) Fellowship

McNair Scholars Program

NEW JERSEY

Cooper Medical School of Rowan University Premedical Urban Leaders Summer Enrichment Program (PULSE)

Health Career Connection Comprehensive Summer Internship Program

Northeast Regional Alliance (NERA) MEDPREP Program

Rutgers University Project L/earn

Rutgers Summer Undergraduate Research Program in Neuroscience (NeuroSURP)

Robert Wood Johnson Medical School Academic Enrichment Programs

Robert Wood Johnson Graduate School of Biomedical Sciences Undergraduate Summer

Research Experience

Robert Wood Johnson Biomedical Careers Program (BCP)

Northeast Regional Alliance MedPrep Scholars Program

NEW YORK

Albert Einstein College of Medicine of Yeshiva University Hispanic Center of Excellence

Summer Undergraduate Mentorship Program

University at Buffalo School of Dental Medicine and Seneca Nation Health System: Native

American Pre-Dental Gateway Program

Columbia University Medical Center Summer Program for Under-Represented Students

(SPURS)

Zucker Pipeline Program (ZPP) at the Donald and Barbara Zucker School of Medicine at

Hofstra/Northwell

Health Career Connection Comprehensive Summer Internship Program

New York University School of Medicine Sackler Institute of Graduate Biomedical Sciences Summer Undergraduate Research Program (SURP)

State University of New York (SUNY) Downstate Medical Center (Multiple programs available)

Summer of Translational Aging Research for Undergraduates (STAR U) at Columbia University

University of Rochester Medical Center Summer Undergraduate Research Fellowship

Weill Medical College of Cornell University The Travelers Summer Research Fellowship Program for Premedical Students

Weill Medical College of Cornell University Weill Cornell/ Rockefeller/ Sloan-Kettering Gateways to the Laboratory Program

Weill Medical College of Cornell University The ACCESS Summer Minority Research Program

NORTH CAROLINA

East Carolina University Brody School of Medicine Summer Program for Future Doctors

Health Career Connection Comprehensive Summer Internship Program

The University of North Carolina at Chapel Hill Medical Education Development Program (MED)

NORTH DAKOTA

University of North Dakota School of Medicine and Health Sciences Indians into Medicine

OHIO

Case Western Reserve University Schools of Medicine and Dental Medicine Heart, Lung, and Blood Minority Research Training Program

Ohio University of Osteopathic Medicine Summer Scholars Program

Ohio University Heritage College of Osteopathic Medicine Summer Undergraduate Research Fellowship (SURF) program

University of Cincinnati College of Medicine Summer Undergraduate Research Fellowships (SURF)

OKLAHOMA

University of Oklahoma Health Sciences Center Headlands Indian Health Careers Program

OREGON

Oregon Health and Science University Equity Summer Research Program

PENNSYLVANIA

University of Pennsylvania The Undergraduate Student Scholars Program NIH Center for Molecular Studies in Digestive and Liver Disease

University of Pennsylvania Undergraduate Clinical Scholars Program

University of Pittsburgh School of Medicine Summer Undergraduate Research Program

TENNESSEE

St. Jude Children's Research Hospital Pediatric Oncology Education (POE) Program

Vanderbilt University Minority Summer Research Program

TEXAS

Texas A&M College of Dentistry SPEP Collegiate II Program

University of North Texas Health Science Center McNair Scholars Program

University of North Texas Health Science Center Summer Multicultural Advanced Research Training (SMART)

University of Texas Health Science Center at San Antonio Summer Programs for Undergraduates

VIRGINIA

Virginia Commonwealth University Summer Academic Enrichment Program (SAEP)

University of Virginia School of Medicine Summer Research Internship Program

WASHINGTON

University of Washington Health Sciences Center STAR Program

WISCONSIN

Marquette University College Science Enrichment Program (CSEP)

Medical College of Wisconsin Multicultural Summer Research Training Program

PROGRAMS IN DENTISTRY

University of California Los Angeles David Geffen Schools of Medicine and Dentistry PREP

Summer Health Professions Education Program

Southern Illinois University School of Medicine Medical/ Dental Education Preparatory Program (MEDPREP)

Baylor College of Dentistry Summer Pre-Dental Enrichment Program

Harvard School of Dental Medicine: Bridge to Dental School (10-week summer program)

PROGRAMS IN OPTOMETRY

University of California, Berkeley Optometry Opto-Camp

Illinois College of Optometry Focus on Your Future Summer Program

State University of New York (SUNY) State College of Optometry Collegiate Science and Technology Entry Program (CSTEP)

The Ohio State University Improving Diversity in Optometric Careers

PROGRAMS IN PHARMACY

Campbell University Healthcare Professionals Readiness & Enrichment Program (H-PREP)

Keck Graduate Institute Pre-Pharmacy Enrichment Summer Program (PrEP)

University at Buffalo Pharmacy Summer Institute

University of Illinois at Chicago College of Pharmacy Summer Pharmacy Institute

University of Illinois at Chicago College of Pharmacy Summer Undergraduate Research Fellowship (SURF)

University of Kansas Undergraduate Research Program

Purdue University Undergraduate Summer Research Fellowships

Virginia Commonwealth University Summer Academic Enrichment Program (SAEP)

PROGRAMS IN VETERNINARY MEDICINE

Woods Hole Oceanographic Institution Minority Fellow Program

University of Pennsylvania Veterinary Exploration Through Science (VETS)

MD/PHD PROGRAMS

University of Alabama at Birmingham Summer in Biological Sciences (SIBS) Undergraduate Research Program

University of California San Diego Summer Undergraduate Research Program (SURF)

University of Cincinnati Physician Scientist Summer Undergraduate Research Fellowship

University of Iowa Summer Undergraduate MSTP Research Program

University of Michigan Undergraduate Summer Research Programs

University of Minnesota Medical School Twin Cities Life Sciences Summer Undergraduate Research Programs

University of Nebraska Medical Center MD/PhD Summer Undergraduate Research Program

NIH-AMGEN Scholars Program

The Ohio State University SUCCESS Program

Washington University in St. Louis BioMedRAP/AMGEN Scholars

Weill Cornell/Rockefeller/Sloan-Kettering Tri-Institutional MD-PhD Program

OTHER PROGRAMS

American Indian Science and Engineering Society

Health Career Connection Comprehensive Summer Internship Program

National Institute of Health Summer Internship Program (STEP-UP)

Summer Research Early Identification Program (SR-EIP)

Youth Health Equity Model of Practice (YHEMOP) Summer Program

Minority Student Pipeline Programs

In order to break down the barriers that prevent many minorities from choosing medicine, the Student National Medical Association's pipeline programs and the Pipeline Mentoring Institute (PMI) were established to improve study skills, improve test-taking skills, and expose students to health careers. To learn more about SNMA, visit www.snma.org/ programs.php. The following are the pipeline programs that have helped thousands of premedical students achieve success in medical school admissions:

- **Pre-medical Minority Enrichment and Development (PMED):** This is a mentoring program in which SNMA members assist premedical minority students in preparing for medical school. The program includes pre-medical conferences, clinical skill workshops, medical student panels, and medical school resources.

- **Minority Association of Pre-medical Students (MAPS):** More than 100 colleges and universities nationwide have SNMA MAPS chapters that participate in local, regional, and national events. Nationally recognized as associate members, MAPS members are eligible for most SNMA national and regional benefits. The chapters are self-governing in accordance with SNMA regional and national bylaws.

- **Brotherhood Alliance for Science Education (BASE):** This program aims to increase the recruitment, admission, and retention of minority males into medicine. BASE seeks to unite minority males around common goals and build relationships that foster a sense of brotherhood among minority males. Among its goals are mentorship, community service, and motivation for worthwhile and attainable goals.

- **Health Careers Exploration Program (HCEP):** Students participate in seminars and problem-based learning sessions. There are opportunities for shadowing and exploring career paths in medicine as well as learning critical thinking skills.

- **Males in Medicine:** Freshman males participate in a four-day, three-night summer outreach conference at Penn State College of Medicine, where there are introduced to life at the medical college from admissions to residency match.

- **Short-Term Educational Program for Underrepresented Persons (STEP-UP):** Students conduct basic or clinical research with experienced faculty during a 10-week summer program in Hershey. Focus areas include diabetes, nutrition and obesity, and digestive, kidney, and hematological diseases.

- **Summer Undergraduate Research Internship Program (SURIP):** Students who have completed at least 2 years of college work in a basic or clinical laboratory in Hershey for 10 weeks.

Some Final Suggestions for Minority Students

Currently, minority applicants have a much better acceptance rate than they did twenty years earlier. Both application and admission trends are up, and interest in medicine is stronger than ever. However, many bright minority students are running into roadblocks because they're not as prepared as they should be. The problem often lies not in their qualifications but in the social hurdles that many minority students still must overcome on the way to a career in medicine.

Because of financial impacts, increasing numbers of minorities below the poverty line face a much tougher road on their way to medical school. Minority youngsters are more likely to attend elementary and high schools in areas of poverty characterized by low academic performance, discipline problems, crimes, low levels of parental involvement, and less qualified and unmotivated teachers. The cumulative impact of these factors begins to show up in lower educational achievement and takes its toll by about age ten.

Minority students, especially in predominately white schools, are sometimes placed into vocational courses or in low-track classes where they're not intellectually challenged, where expectations are lower, and where the message is sent that they cannot aspire to higher scholastic achievement. Add rising tuition rates, low graduation rates from high school, lack of role models, and increasing interest in other professions such as business and computer technology, and you have fewer minorities pursuing medicine as a career than the population demands.

The good news is that medical schools are actively pursuing minority students. Premedical programs are also serious about increasing minority applications and are focusing on ways to improve academic skills and MCAT scores, providing role models and mentors, and increasing financial assistance. However, minority students cannot assume that they have an advantage just because they're in an underrepresented group. Medical school admission is tough, and you still must have the grades, the MCAT scores, and the extracurricular activities to be competitive. Besides the areas already mentioned, here are some final suggestions minority students can use to improve their chances of being successful medical school applicants.

- Minority students who participate in high school or college science and math programs are more likely to be accepted into medical school than non-participants. College-level enrichment programs that have proven particularly valuable in improving medical school acceptance rates are educational programs that provide a summer laboratory experience. You need to take advantage of any opportunity that will enhance your academic credentials.
- Too few minority high school and college students take advanced science and math courses. Math and science skills directly affect performance on standardized tests and are gatekeepers to higher education. Programs that include MCAT preparation, for example, can improve test scores significantly. This alone could mean the difference between acceptance and rejection. One of the biggest trouble spots minority students have is the MCAT. Preparation courses are beneficial because they teach you how to take the MCAT exam.
- Unless a student gets serious from day one, college may be too late to improve academic skills and knowledge of science and math. Therefore, preparation should really begin in high school. According to statistics, a student's MCAT performance could be predicted accurately from scores on the SAT taken in the last year of high school. This finding suggests that, to maximize your chances for success, you need to take high school seriously.
- Minority students who apply to five or more medical schools and who receive help with the application process are more likely to be accepted than those who do not. Applying to more schools will increase the chances that your qualifications, credentials, and background will match the admissions criteria of a given school.
- Non-academic factors such as poor guidance counseling and insufficient career information contribute greatly to the loss of minorities from the medical applicant pool. If your school does not have a good guidance counselor, or it lacks information, don't be afraid to go somewhere else for advice. Also, never assume that your counselor knows what is best for you or even that he or she has your best interests at heart. Dr. Benjamin Carson, the world-famous black neurosurgeon and presidential

candidate, was told by his advisor that he was not smart enough to be a doctor. Dr. Carson was
smart enough to ignore that advice!

- Having minority physicians as role models and mentors is key to many minority students' success. Role models and mentors provide valuable standards of achievement, inspire career choices, and lay out avenues for upward mobility. You need to find a role model or mentor from medical school, from your community, or your hospital. These role models will help you compensate for the isolation you'll often encounter in academic and professional settings where you'll no doubt be underrepresented. More than anything else, your mentor will encourage you when things get tough, and give you the needed inspiration you need to keep going.

  Some thirty years ago, I had the privilege of meeting Dr. Benjamin Carson who, at the age of 38, was already the chief of pediatric surgery at Johns Hopkins University School of Medicine. He'd spoken at NC A&T State University to students interested in health careers. The message he brought was simple: "Anyone can do anything they want if they set their mind to it and are prepared to work hard to achieve their goals." He went on to say that "Blacks and other minorities have every opportunity to pursue health careers and can rise as far as they are willing to go," and that "it doesn't matter what color you are; if you're willing to work hard and become the best you can be, people will beat down your door to give you an opportunity to succeed."

From a Detroit ghetto, where he almost destroyed his life, to Yale University, and finally to medical school, Dr. Carson became one of only a handful of black neurosurgeons in the world. The reason: he never stopped believing that he could do whatever he set out to do. You, too, can follow that example and achieve your goal of medical school if you're willing to work harder than you've ever worked before. With enough desire and determination, your chances of gaining admission to medical school are much better than you think.

Since 1975, when minorities represented just 8 percent of the total student body, minority enrollment in U.S. medical schools has been rising steadily. But in a changing and more diverse healthcare environment, it's not enough. The AAMC and its members have stepped up their efforts to attract more African American and other minorities to pursue careers in medicine; and now, more than ever, you have a real opportunity to become part of a career that others only dream of.

CHAPTER 10

FOREIGN MEDICAL EDUCATION

One of the last options you might want to consider, only if you've been unsuccessful for several years in gaining admission to a U.S. medical school, is to apply to one or more foreign or offshore medical schools. There's really no way to determine how many students choose this option each year, but the numbers have been steadily increasing because of the record number of applicants vying for limited space in U.S. medical programs. The problem is, with language barriers, varied curricula, cultural differences, and sometimes inferior faculty members, it's difficult to know what you're getting yourself into and how successful you'll be once you come back to the United States. Students can spend thousands of dollars their first year, only to find out that the school they chose is not all it promised to be.

There are some excellent medical schools throughout the world, especially in Western Europe. A few of them even offer their curriculums entirely in English (the Philippines and some in the Caribbean, for example), which makes life for students much easier. Many European medical schools, however, only accept applications from their own citizens and, therefore, you must do your research and plan accordingly. Canadian medical schools are not considered "foreign" by the AAMC but they accept only a very few American students each year. It's much harder, even for an outstanding candidate, to get into any Canadian school.

Before you decide on applying to any foreign medical school, you should seriously consider other options like waiting a year or two while you improve your academic and non-academic credentials, or applying to osteopathic schools, especially if you're interested in primary care. The government accounting office (GAO) has visited many foreign schools and found that, unlike U.S. medical school programs, they differ considerably. In the GAO's opinion, none of the foreign medical schools offer a medical education comparable to that available in the United States due to deficiencies in admission requirements, equipment, faculty, curriculum, and clinical training. Although it's difficult to judge foreign schools in all these areas, one of the most serious deficiencies was the lack of adequate clinical training facilities.

Pros and Cons of Applying to a Foreign Medical School

Each year, thousands of students decide that they would rather begin medical training, regardless of where it is, rather than wait and reapply to U.S. medical schools or retake the MCAT. For some students, it works out; for others, it's a nightmare. It all depends on the quality of the program and how well the school prepares you for the medical boards. Some Caribbean medical schools are new, so their programs have not been well established. Others do not have particularly good reputations for student success. Students must do their research and make sure that whatever school they apply to is reputable. Here are some pros and cons:

Pros:

Acceptance rates are much higher at foreign medical schools, especially in the Caribbean, than they are in the United States.

Caribbean medical schools are much more lenient when considering grades and MCAT scores. Students who graduate with GPAs of 3.0 and average MCAT scores have a better chance of admission.

Students at Caribbean medical schools typically do their last two-year rotations in U.S. hospitals, most commonly in the New York area. This is an advantage when applying for U.S. residency programs.

Many of the faculty members are non-practicing physicians and place an emphasis on teaching, which means they're available more.

Cons:

Grading systems can vary from school to school, with many Caribbean medical schools still maintaining a traditional A-F system. By contrast, most U.S. medical schools rely on the Honors/Pass/Fail grading system, which places less stress on an already competitive school environment.

Teaching quality can be highly variable. Some schools have many visiting professors who only come to the country on vacation and teach a class for 2-4 weeks.

Living in a different country with a new language, different culture, and lack of amenities can be challenging.

Matching to a U.S. residency program can be more difficult. Competition for residencies is increasing, and graduates of foreign medical schools are much less successful in getting those residencies, especially in popular specialties. For example, while almost 95 percent of U.S. medical school graduates matched into a residency program, less than 50 percent of foreign medical school graduates matched. Because there are more graduates than residency slots, preference is given to U.S. graduates, and it will soon be nearly impossible for a foreign medical school graduate to get a residency of his or her choice.

New York's sixteen medical schools are fighting to make it harder for foreign schools to use New York hospitals for their clinical rotations. The changes, if approved, could close some of the Caribbean medical schools because their islands lack the hospitals and clinical facilities to provide the hands-on training a doctor needs to be licensed in the United States.

Accreditation of Foreign Medical Schools

The Purpose of the National Committee on Foreign Medical Education and Accreditation (NCFMEA) is to review the standards used by foreign countries to accredit medical schools and to determine whether those standards are comparable to standards used to accredit medical schools in the United States. The NCFMEA does not review or accredit individual foreign medical schools. It only reviews the standards a foreign country uses to accredit its medical schools. The request by a foreign country for review by the NCFMEA is voluntary. For more information about NCFMEA, visit their website.

The countries listed below have been reviewed by the NCFMEA and found to use standards to accredit their medical schools that are comparable to the standards used to accredit medical schools in the United States. Next to the country are the dates on which the commission made their decision of comparability, along with the agency that accredits medical schools in that country.

Antigua and Barbuda (10/13, 2020) – Caribbean Accreditation Authority

Australia (2/95, 3/01, 9/07, 9/09, 4/17, 2020) - Australian Medical Council

(Note: The Australian Medical Council also accredits medical schools in New Zealand under the terms of an agreement with that country.)

Barbados (9/16, 2022) - Caribbean Accreditation Authority

Canada (2/95, 3/01, 3/09, 10/15, 2021) - Committee on Accreditation of Canadian Medical Schools

Cayman Islands (9/02, 9/03, 9/04, 3/09, 10/15, 2021) - Accreditation Commission on Colleges of Medicine

Czech Republic (3/98, 9/04, 10/11, 2021) - Czech Republic Accreditation Commission

Dominica (10/97, 3/01, 3/07, 9/18, 2020) - Ministry of Health & Social Security and the Dominica Medical Board

Dominican Republic (10/97, 3/04, 4/13, 2021) - National Council of Higher Education, Science and Technology

Grenada (9/96, 3/03, 3/07, 4/16, 2021) - Grenada Ministry of Health, Social Security, The Environment, and Ecclesiastical Relations in conjunction with the New York State Department of Education's Office of the Professions

Hungary (3/97, 3/03, 10/11, 9/18, 2020) - Hungarian Accreditation Committee

Ireland (3/97, 9/03, 9/09, 9/18, 2020) - Irish Medical Council

Israel (9/99, 9/08, 4/19, 2022) - Council for Higher Education

Mexico (10/97, 3/04, 4/14, 2020) - Mexican Board for the Accreditation of Medical Education

Netherlands (3/98, 9/07, 4/14, 2020) - Netherlands Flemish Accreditation Organization

Poland (10/97, 9/03, 10/11, 9/17, 2020) - Ministry of Health/Accreditation Committee of Polish Universities of Medical Sciences

Saint Kitts and Nevis (4/12, 4/19, 2022) - Accreditation Commission on Colleges of Medicine

Saint Vincent and the Grenadines (9/16, 2022) - Caribbean Accreditation Authority

St. Maarten (3/98, 3/04, 10/11, 9/18, 2021) - Accreditation Commission on Colleges of Medicine

Taiwan (3/02, 3/09, 9/17, 2021) - Taiwan Medical Accreditation Council

United Kingdom (9/96, 9/01, 3/09, 4/17, 2023) - General Medical Council

When applying to any foreign medical school, it's important to make sure that 1) it's accredited and listed in the International Medical Education Directory (IMED) because if it's not, you won't be eligible for certification to practice in the U.S., and 2) it meets the same standards used to accredit U.S. medical schools. It doesn't make much sense to pay more than $100,000 to attend a subpar medical school that has a poor record of success.

Caribbean Medical Programs

One of the main reasons that U.S. citizens are choosing medical schools in the Caribbean is that many have a similar accreditation system to U.S. medical schools. Furthermore, their curricula and training parallel medical schools here because graduating students must still pass the United States Licensing Examination once they return. Most Caribbean medical schools require 90 credit hours from an accredited university, although some do not require an undergraduate degree. A few do not require the MCAT. The average GPA of applicants is 3.3, but students with GPAs of less than 3.0 have gained admission. MCAT scores are typically less than they are for students applying to U.S. medical schools.

There are over 60 medical schools in the Caribbean, categorized as either regional or offshore, but only about 40 are accredited. Regional medical schools train students to practice in the country or region where the school is located. Offshore medical schools train students from the United States and Canada who will return home after graduation. Students at offshore medical schools spend the first two years of basic sciences in the Caribbean and then complete their clinical clerkships at teaching hospitals in the United States, primarily in the New York area. The following is a list of popular and accredited Caribbean medical schools, along with their locations and year they were established:

All American Institute of Medical Sciences
Location: Jamaica
Year Established: 2011

All Saints University College of Medicine
Location: Saint Vincent and the Grenadines
Year Established: 2011

University of the West Indies Faculty of Medicine
Location: Barbados
Year Established: 1967

American International Medical University
Location: Saint Lucia
Year Established: 2007

American University of Antigua College of Medicine
Location: Antigua
Year Established: 2004

American University of Barbados School of Medicine
Location: Barbados
Year Established: 2011

University of the West Indies Faculty of Medicine
Location: Barbados
Year Established: 1967

American University of St Vincent School of Medicine
Location: Saint Vincent and the Grenadines
Year Established: 2012

University of the West Indies Faculty of Medicine
Location: Barbados
Year Established: 1967

American University of the Caribbean School of Medicine
Location: St Maarten
Year Established: 1978

American University School of Medicine Aruba
Location: Aruba
Year Established: 2011

Atlantic University School of Medicine
Location: Saint Lucia
Year Established: 2010

Aureus University School of Medicine
Location: Aruba
Year Established: 2004

Avalon University School of Medicine
Location: Curacao
Year Established: 2003

Caribbean Medical University School of Medicine
Location: Curacao
Year Established: 2007

Central American Health Sciences University, Belize Medical College
Location: Belize
Year Established: 1996

International American University, College of Medicine
Location: Saint Lucia
Year Established: 2003

International University of Health Sciences School of Medicine
Location: Saint Kitts and Nevis
Year Established: 1998

John F. Kennedy University School of Medicine
Location: Curacao
Year Established: 2014

Medical University of the Americas
Location: Saint Kitts and Nevis
Year Established: 1998

New York Medical University
Location: Curacao
Year Established: 2017

Ross University School of Medicine
Location: Barbados
Year Established: 1978

Saba University School of Medicine
Location: Saba (Netherlands)
Year Established: 1994

Spartan Health Sciences University School of Medicine
Location: Saint Lucia
Year Established: 1980

St George's University
Location: Grenada
Year Established: 1977

St Martinus University Faculty of Medicine
Location: Curacao
Year Established: 2000

St Matthew's University School of Medicine
Location: Grand Cayman
Year Established: 2002

Trinity School of Medicine
Location: Saint Vincent and the Grenadines
Year Established: 2008

University of Guyana
Location: Guyana
Year Established: 1985

University of Health Sciences Antigua School of Medicine
Location: Antigua and Barbuda
Year Established: 1983

University of Medicine and Health Sciences - St Kitts
Location: Saint Kitts and Nevis
Year Established: 2008

University of Saint Eustatius School of Medicine
Location: Saint Eustatius (Netherlands)
Year Established:

University of Science, Arts and Technology College of Medicine
Location: Montserrat
Year Established: 2003

University of the West Indies Faculty of Medicine
Location: Barbados
Year Established: 1967

University of the West Indies Faculty of Medicine at St. Augustine
Location: Trinidad and Tobago
Year Established: 1967

University of the West Indies Faculty of Medicine
Location: Barbados
Year Established: 1967

Washington University of Health and Science
Location: Belize
Year Established: 2005

Xavier University School of Medicine at Aruba
Location: Aruba (Netherlands)
Year Established: 2004

Other Medical School Options Abroad

None of the foreign medical schools examined by the government accounting office had access to the same range of clinical facilities and numbers and variety of patients as United States programs. Many of these schools are in poor countries that sometimes lack modern conveniences. Caribbean schools have been especially suspect in recent years because of curriculum deficiencies and poor teaching facilities.

Students sometimes choose Western European medical schools for several reasons: many European medical schools have good track records in offering a quality medical education, and some offer 6-year programs in which students can begin studying medicine right after high school. During the last few years, however, a more formal and stringent selection process has become necessary due to the increasing complexity of medicine and the increasing numbers of both national and international applicants. Here are some interesting facts about medical schools in Europe and what they use to select their medical students. The list is by no means complete, but it should give you an idea of what you would be up against when considering this path.

Many countries have special citizenry requirements for entrance into their medical schools, so applicants need to check with the school to see if they even allow U.S. citizens to apply.

In almost every country, the average age of candidates at the time of selection is 21, which contrasts with the United States medical school average age of 25. There's more of a tendency for European medial schools to take age into consideration than it is for medical schools in the United States.

In general, there's a growing trend to admit more women applicants. The current rate is somewhere between 30 and 40 percent, compared to 50 percent or more in the United States.

Different countries often have quite different entrance requirements. For example, in Germany, 60 percent of admissions are based on scores of undergraduate exams. In the Netherlands, entrance is based on overall science scores on the final secondary school examinations. In Sweden, grades obtained during the final years of secondary school are taken into consideration.

Because of limited space and facilities, some countries have lottery systems for admitting students who were not accepted immediately.

Some countries make special allowances for students who've served in the armed forces or who have participated in a medically related activity or job.

By far, the greatest numbers of students apply to Caribbean medical schools. However, there are some excellent medical schools in other countries that accept U.S. citizens, and some are even affiliated with U.S. institutions. Here are some popular medical schools that have been successful in graduating students:

Medical Schools in Israel

There are five medical schools in Israel that all follow the European six-year model: Technion Medical School in Haifa, Ben Gurion University of the Negev, Tel Aviv University, and the Hebrew University in Jerusalem. In 2009, Tel Aviv University introduced a four-year program for students with a bachelor's degree in biological sciences. Technion Medical School, Ben Gurion University, and Tel Aviv University offer 4-year MD programs for American students who have American college degrees and have taken the MCAT. All schools in Israel are rated as excellent.

Bar-Ilan University: Based in the Galilee, it has teaching hospitals in Nahariyah, Nazareth, Safed, and Tiberias.

Ben-Gurion Medical School: Collaborating with Columbia University Medical Center in New York, it has teaching hospitals in Beersheva, Ashkelon, and Eilat. It also has an international medical school for foreign students with an emphasis on global health.

Hebrew University, Hadassah Medical School: With teaching hospitals in Jerusalem and Rehovot, it also runs a parallel program with an emphasis on military medicine and where students are admitted directly from high school.

Technion, Rappaport Medical School: With its main teaching hospitals in Haifa and Afula, it also has a parallel program for graduate level foreign students.

Tel Aviv University Medical School: The university has main teaching hospitals in Tel Aviv, Ramat Gan, Tikva, and Holon, and allows foreign students into a parallel program.

Medical Schools in Ireland

Irish medical schools are a popular choice for applicants because of their good reputation and their connections with schools in the United States. The Atlantic Bridge Program is a cultural diversity program that allows a small number of Canadian and U.S. students to study medicine at an Irish University. Approximately 200 North American students are accepted each year.

The 4-year program requires an undergraduate degree and the MCAT, the 5-year program requires only an undergraduate degree, and the 6-year program requires a secondary education. All students must also submit a personal statement, two letters of recommendation, a resume, and transcripts.

Students can apply to all eight Irish medical schools using one common application and submitting only one set of documents (transcripts, letters of reference etc.). After graduation from the Atlantic Bridge Program, students have the choice of entering postgraduate residency training in the USA, in Canada, or abroad.

Medical Schools in Australia

There are currently twenty-one medical programs that accept applications from international students for approximately 400 places. Australian medical schools usually have a single intake of students in February/March. Application for the following year's intake opens early in the year, so it's important to know the application closing dates for the various universities in order not to miss out. GPA and MCAT requirements are typically lower than they are for U.S. medical schools, with the minimum GPA being about 2.7.

The University of Queensland Medical Degree Program in Brisbane accepts the most applicants. This program is designed for U.S. students or permanent residents and provides students two years of rotations in the United States at the Ochsner Clinical School in New Orleans. Students complete their first two years studying the basic medical sciences at The University of Queensland's School of Medicine and then complete their clinical rotations in New Orleans. Ochsner Health System is a multi-specialty healthcare delivery system that includes seven hospitals and over 35 health centers located throughout Southeast Louisiana. Medical students work alongside students from Tulane University and the University of Louisiana School of Medicine, who also pursue clinical studies through the Ochsner Health System.

Medical Schools in Poland

Poland offers more medical programs in English than any other Eastern European country. It also has the most involved admissions process with the most steps. Several of the schools require the MCAT or a specialty examination in chemistry, biology, and physics (given by the university). The medical programs available in English are:

Medical Academy of Bialystok, 4- and 6-year programs

Medical University in Bydgoszcz, 6-year program

Medical Academy of Gdansk, 6-year program

Medical University of Lodz, 4-year program

Medical University of Lublin, 4- and 6-year programs

Jagiellonian University Medical College, 4- and 6-year programs

Pomeranian Academy of Medicine, 6-year program

Poznan School of Medicine, 4- and 6-year programs

Medical University of Silesia, 4- and 6-year programs

Medical University of Warsaw, 4- and 6-year programs

Wroclaw Medical University, 6-year medical program

The quality of programs in other, non-Polish, Eastern European medical schools varies significantly, and most don't offer curricula in English. When considering Eastern European medical schools, make sure that you carefully consider their reputations.

Educational Commission for Foreign Medical Graduates (ECFMG)

Established in 1956, ECFMG assesses whether international medical graduates (IMGs) are qualified to enter residency or fellowship programs in the United States. The commission defines an IMG as any U.S. citizen who has received an M.D. from a medical school located outside the United States and Canada. ECFMG certification is also required to take step 3 of the medical licensing examination (USMLE). This ensures that IMGs have met the minimum standards for patient care. As recently as 2020, IMGs accounted for more than 25% of the total U.S. physician population; and with the anticipated shortage of doctors over the next decade, that number is expected to increase.

Before IMGs can practice in the United States, they must go through several steps to evaluate and assess their medical competence. ECFMG certification is only step one in the process, and a significant number of IMGs do not meet one or more of the requirements. For example, a student can graduate from medical school but not pass all the examinations required. And though a student is certified, it does not guarantee a residency position. To obtain a license to practice in the U.S., IMGs must complete the following requirements:

- Complete all coursework, clinical rotations, and other requirements necessary for a medical degree.

- Obtain a medical degree from a medical school listed in the International Medical Education Directory (IMED) and have been awarded credit for at least four academic years by the medical school listed in IMED.

- Pass the licensing examination (USMLE). This includes passing performance on medical science and clinical skills examinations: Step 1, Step 2 Clinical Knowledge (CK), and Step 3 Clinical Skills (CS). Only students who have attended medical schools listed in the IMED are eligible.

- Be certified by ECFMG. To be eligible, IMGs must submit an application before they apply for examination, satisfy the medical science examination requirement (USMLE Step 1 and Step 2 Clinical Knowledge), satisfy the clinical skills requirement (USMLE Step 2 Clinical Skills), and meet their school's medical education credential requirement.

- Obtain a position as a resident or fellow in a U.S. graduate education program (GME).

- Complete the required period of training in a GME.

- Fulfill any additional licensure requirements.

As you can see, students graduating from foreign medical schools have some very hard work to do before they can practice medicine in the United States. This is considered a good thing because it ensures that the quality of medical care is not compromised and that graduates are well-qualified to care for patients. It may seem like a lot of work, but if your goal is to become a physician, and you've run out of options, this could be a viable alternative.

Choosing the Best Foreign Medical School

If you have not been accepted to a United States medical school, I would recommend that you try several more times before opting for the foreign school route. Even though there were more than 50,000 applicants vying for U.S. medical schools last year, there were approximately 24,000 openings, an acceptance rate of about 40 percent. That means between one-third and one-half of all applicants get in somewhere. Some students simply apply to the wrong medical schools or they need to do more work on their qualifications.

Chances are, if you plan a little better, improve your academic standing, and increase your participation in extracurricular activities, you'll become a successful candidate the second or even third time around. One of the best ways to improve those chances, if your academic credentials are not great, is to establish residence in a state with several medical schools. The more medical schools you apply to, the better the odds are. By becoming a state resident, gaining a year's work experience, and enhancing your extracurricular activities, you should be able to get into one of the state medical colleges.

If all else fails, you must still look very carefully and intelligently at your choices of foreign schools. The drop-out rate for non-foreign students at these colleges is quite high. Almost 70 percent of first year medical students leave before or after completed their freshman year. And for those who do make it through four years, there's no guarantee that they'll be able to get into residency programs.

The reasons for high failure rates vary, but they have a lot to do with how students choose the school. Most students do not get enough information about the school to make a good judgment. Consequently, they waste their time and money on a poor education that will not even allow them to come back to the States. You cannot imagine the number of bad medical schools that prey on desperate premedical students who'll pay any price to get admitted and become doctors. These programs count on that. Unfortunately, the probability that these students will receive a first-rate medical education is low. Here are some questions to ask yourself before deciding to apply to any foreign medical school:

Is the medical school accredited and listed in International Medical Education Directory (IMED)? If not, then you're basically throwing your money away.

What language is the curriculum taught in? Are you fluent in that language, or will you be fluent once you begin? If you think medical school is tough, you've not seen anything till you try it in another language.

Are the clinical facilities comparable to those in the United States? Much of a medical education is not classroom time but clinical time. Unless a medical school can offer you quality exposure, you're not going to get the proper training required to be successful.

Is the coursework and the course load similar to that offered by medical schools in the United States? Compare brochures and catalogues and see for yourself if the foreign school is shortchanging you. If the curriculum seems too easy, or if the coursework does not involve a wide variety of subject matter, it's not a good sign that the program is rigorous enough.

Are the professors full-time faculty members devoted to the program, or are they mostly visiting professors from the United States who go on vacation for a few weeks and teach at the medical school in their spare time?

What is the graduation and failure rate of United States students who've gone to a particular foreign medical school? This will give you a good indication of what to expect. To get the latest results of how U.S. citizens have done on the ECFMG examination, write directly to ECFMG and request the statistics.

Deciding which foreign medical school is best for you will be especially important when you finally try to reenter the United States to practice medicine or to apply to a residency program. How well a medical school prepares you for licensure is critical, and some schools are much better than others in terms of pass rates. To measure how foreign medical schools have stacked up against U.S. medical schools in terms of pass rates on medical licensing exams, the Government Accounting Office (GAO) has looked at ten years of data that included all three steps of the licensing exam. While some students did well, on average they did not fare very well compared to graduates from U.S. medical schools.

	1st Attempt	2nd Attempt	3rd Attempt	4th Attempt
Step 1				
U.S. Medical School Graduate	97%	66%	66%	100%
Foreign Medical School Graduate	64%	42%	41%	27%
Step 2 Clinical Knowledge				
U.S. Medical School Graduate	97%	75%	71%	80%
Foreign Medical School Graduate	72%	48%	52%	29%
Step 2 Clinical Skills				
U.S. Medical School Graduate	98%	95%	100%	NA
Foreign Medical School Graduate	82%	77%	63%	0%
Step 3				
U.S. Medical School Graduate	96%	75%	68%	75%
Foreign Medical School Graduate	71%	54%	56%	23%

Transferring Back to the United States

The goal of any medical student studying abroad is to return to the United States as a third-year student, or to enter a U.S. residency program. Unfortunately, the number of residency openings throughout the United States is less than the number of yearly U.S. medical school graduates. Moreover, with the health care system making every effort to reduce costs, there will be less opportunity for certain residencies in the future. When it comes right down to it, foreign medical school graduates, unless they have studied at one of the top-notch institutions, and even if they had, will usually get last preference.

According to the National Resident Matching Program (NRMP), less than 50 percent of foreign medical school graduates have typically been placed in residency programs compared to 95 percent of U.S. medical school graduates. The most competitive specialties like orthopedics or plastic surgery usually do not consider international graduates at all. To make matters worse, the number of American graduates of foreign medical schools applying for United States residencies has more than tripled recently, reducing further the chances of getting into a residency program. Bottom line: graduating from a foreign medical school is not the way to go if you want to be competitive with U.S. graduates. For this reason, hundreds of students consider transferring back to U.S. medical schools every year.

Unfortunately, the number of third year places in U.S. medical schools is not expected to change much and, so, your chances of transferring into a medical school during your third or fourth year is not very good. Moreover, only a handful of U.S. medical schools even consider foreign transfer applicants, and some schools will only consider U.S. residents of their home state enrolled in a foreign medical school. The AAMC keeps a database of individual school transfer policies, so students can contact them to see which schools consider applicants from universities overseas. In most cases, it's best to contact the individual school for the most current information and policies.

To be considered for transfer, students need to have outstanding academic credentials and must have taken Step 1 of the USMLE and achieved a score above 200. Unofficially, to even be competitive, a foreign medical transfer applicant needs to have higher USMLE scores than a U.S. medical student. During the last few years, the actual number of U.S. citizens admitted as transfer students with advanced standing has declined more than 30 percent. Even passing the exam does not necessarily mean automatic admission to a U.S. medical school.

The process of transferring from a foreign to a U.S. medical school is extremely difficult. Students who choose to study abroad should do so with the expectation that they'll graduate from the foreign medical school but should not assume that it's easier to transfer back to the United States once they have a few years of medical school under their belt. So before applying to any foreign medical school, know what you're getting yourself into and get as much information about the school as possible. It's your future, and only you can decide if this is the right path for you.

CHAPTER 11

FINANCING A MEDICAL EDUCATION

Money can certainly create a lot of stress and anxiety if you're considering medical school but are afraid of what it will cost you. For the 2024 academic year, for example, tuition and fees at public medical schools averaged about $52,000 for in-state students and $65,000 for out-of-state students. For private schools, annual tuition was more than $65,000. Add to those numbers other expenses such as rent and the cost of living and the financial burden can be staggering.

The lack of money, however, does not have to keep you from considering a medical career. Many sources of financial aid are available; some geared specifically toward helping minority or disadvantaged students. But anyone can find sources of financial aid, such as scholarships, grants, loans, and work-study, if he or she is willing to look for them. You should approach financial planning just as you do application and admission planning. The sooner you begin, the more secure you will be in getting the funding you'll need.

Even though medical school is expensive, there's good news. Medical school is the best return on your investment, and no medical school will turn an applicant away because of finances. Many students from poor backgrounds have been successful in medical school, despite the difficulty they faced financially. Like thousands of others, you, too, can get through medical school regardless of your financial position and family background. The best way to ensure that you know about all the possibilities regarding financial aid is to consult the financial aid officer and student services director at the school and to shop around as early as possible for summer job opportunities.

Working While in Medical School

Because of the academic demands placed on medical students, most medical schools discourage employment, full or part-time, during the school year, especially during the first two years of the curriculum. Not all schools frown on part-time work, however; and there are a few that will even assist medical students in finding suitable work, so long as they keep their grades up. Having been affiliated with a medical school, and seeing what medical students go through, I would recommend that a medical student find some sort of financial aid and not even attempt to work.

If accepted to medical school, it will be up to you to find out about financial aid from the school's financial aid department. Contact the financial aid officer soon after you've been notified of your acceptance and request that financial aid applications be sent to you. Normally, financial assistance is based on financial need, but a limited number of schools also offer scholarships, grants, and awards based on demonstrated academic excellence. When you receive applications, complete them as soon as you can and send them in to be processed.

Other sources of financial aid, besides the various awards offered by medical schools, are available to qualified applicants. The sooner you apply and get an award, the sooner you can stop worrying about money and start concentrating on doing well during your first year of medical school. Counseling is readily available at all medical schools, and the qualified staff will ensure that you get some sort of assistance during your four years.

Free Application for Federal Student Aid (FAFSA)

Before you do anything else, the first step in securing financial aid is to go online and complete your Free Application for Federal Student Aid form. As part of the Department of Education, Federal Student Aid is the largest provider of student financial aid in the nation, providing more than $150 billion in federal grants, loans, and work-study funds each year to more than 15 million students paying for college or career school. Many of these, however, such as Pell grants and Federal Supplemental Education Opportunity Grants (FSEOG), are specifically set aside for undergraduate students. As an undergraduate premed student, you would be eligible for every type of financial aid, including grants, scholarships, and loans.

Medical schools use FAFSA to determine if you're eligible for need-based assistance, tuition waivers, or school-sponsored awards other than those exclusively for undergraduate studies. It's important to file the form in January because financial aid is typically awarded on a first-come, first-served basis; so the sooner you submit your application, the better. Once a medical school runs out of financial aid funds, you are out of luck. To learn about the various types of aid and to complete your application online, go to www.fafsa.ed.gov.

Grants and Scholarships Available to Premedical Students

Grants and scholarships, unlike loans, do not have to be repaid once you graduate. While grants are often need-based, scholarships are usually merit-based. They can come from federal or state government, the college or university, or private and non-profit organizations. The following are some of the most common:

- **Pell Grant.** Federal Pell Grants are awarded only to undergraduate students who have not earned a bachelor's or a professional degree. You will not be eligible to receive a Federal Pell Grant if you're incarcerated in a federal or state penal institution or are subject to an involuntary civil commitment upon completion of a period of incarceration for a forcible or non-forcible sexual offense. The amount awarded depends on your financial need, the cost of attending school, your status as a full-time or part-time student, and your plans to attend a college or university for a full academic year or less.

- **Federal Supplemental Educational Opportunity Grant (FSEOG).** To get an FSEOG, your college will determine how much financial need you have. Students who receive Federal Pell Grants and have the most financial need will receive FSEOGs first. The FSEOG program is administered directly by the financial aid office at each participating school and is therefore called "campus-based" aid. Not all schools participate, however. Check with your school's financial aid office in order to find out if the school offers the FSEOG.
- **Iraq and Afghanistan Service Grant.** You would be eligible to receive the Iraq and Afghanistan Service Grant as long as you're not eligible to receive a Federal Pell, you meet the remaining Federal Pell Grant eligibility requirements, your parent or guardian was a member of the U.S. armed forces and died as a result of military service performed in Iraq or Afghanistan after the events of 9/11, and you were under 24 years old or enrolled in college at least part-time at the time of your parent's or guardian's death.
- **National Science and Mathematics Access to Retain Talent Grant (SMART).** This grant is available to undergraduate students who are in their third or fourth year of undergraduate studies. To be eligible for a SMART grant, students must: (1) also be eligible for the Federal Pell Grant, (2) major in life sciences, physical sciences, engineering, mathematics, technology, or computer sciences, and (3) maintain a 3.0 GPA in their major.
- **Scholarships for Disadvantaged Students (SDS).** The Scholarships for Disadvantaged Students program provides funds to schools and not to individuals. In turn, the schools make scholarships to full-time, financially needy students from disadvantaged backgrounds, regardless of race, enrolled in health professions programs. You are eligible to apply for this scholarship at any school that participates in the Scholarships for Disadvantaged Students program if you are from a disadvantaged background as defined by the U.S. Department of Health and Human Services, and are a United States citizen, national, or a lawful permanent resident of the United States or the District of Columbia, the Commonwealths of Puerto Rico or the Marianas Islands, the Virgin Islands, Guam, the American Samoa, the Trust Territory of the Pacific Islands, the Republic of Palau, the Republic of the Marshall Islands and the Federated State of Micronesia. Check with your school's financial aid office to see if they participate in the program.
- **Janelia Undergraduate Scholars Program.** This scholars program gives outstanding undergraduate students the opportunity to experience research for 10

weeks during the summer in the Washington, DC area. Students receive a $5,000 stipend and work on a wide range of scientific research projects. To learn more, visit http://www.janelia.org/student-programs/undergraduate-program.

Loans Available to both Premedical and Medical Students

There are several types of loans available to undergraduate and/or medical students. Unlike grants and scholarships, loans must be repaid. Check with your school to see if they participate in any type of loan program. Here are some of the more common loans available:

- **Direct Subsidized Loans**. These loans are available to undergraduate students enrolled at least half-time at a school that participates in the Direct Loan Program and in a program that leads to a degree or certificate awarded by the school. Your school determines the amount you can borrow, and the amount may not exceed your financial need. The U.S. Department of Education pays the interest on a Direct Subsidized Loan while you are in school at least half-time, for the first six months after you leave school, and during a period of deferment (a postponement of loan payments).
- **Direct Unsubsidized Loans**. These loans are available to both undergraduate and graduate students (medical students), and there is no requirement to demonstrate financial need. You are not required to show financial need to receive a Direct Unsubsidized Loan. Your school determines the amount you can borrow based on your cost of attendance and other financial aid you receive. You are responsible for paying the interest on the loan during all periods.
- **Plus Loans**. These loans are federal loans that graduate or medical school students and parents of dependent undergraduate students can use to help pay education expenses. The U.S. Department of Education makes Direct PLUS Loans to eligible borrowers through schools participating in the Direct Loan Program. To receive a Direct PLUS Loan, you must be a graduate or professional degree student enrolled at least half-time at an eligible school in a program leading to a degree or certificate, or be the parent (biological, adoptive, or in some cases, stepparent) of a dependent undergraduate student enrolled at least half-time at a participating school, and meet the general eligibility requirements for federal student aid. If you are borrowing on behalf of your child, your child must also meet these requirements.
- **Federal Perkins Loan Program**. Loans made through the Federal Perkins Loan Program, often called Perkins Loans, are low-interest federal student loans for both undergraduate and graduate students with exceptional financial need. Not all schools participate in the Federal Perkins Loan Program, so you should check with your school's financial aid office to see if your school participates. Since your school is the lender, you will make your payments to the school that made your loan or your school's loan servicer. Funds depend on your financial need and the availability of funds at your college.

- **Health Professions Student Loan (HPSL).** The Health Professions Student Loan program provides long-term, low interest rate loans to full-time, financially needy students to pursue a degree in dentistry, optometry, pharmacy, podiatric medicine, or veterinary medicine. You're eligible to apply for this loan if you are a citizen, national, or a lawful permanent resident of the United States or the District of Columbia, the Commonwealths of Puerto Rico or the Marianas Islands, the Virgin Islands, Guam, the American Samoa, the Trust Territory of the Pacific Islands, the Republic of Palau, the Republic of the Marshall Islands and the Federated State of Micronesia. Check with your school to see if they participate in the program.
- **Loans for Disadvantaged Students (LDS).** The Loans for Disadvantaged Students program provides long-term, low-interest rate loans to full-time, financially needy students from disadvantaged backgrounds, to pursue a degree in allopathic medicine, osteopathic medicine, dentistry, optometry, podiatric medicine, pharmacy or veterinary medicine. Participating schools are responsible for selecting loan recipients, making reasonable determinations of need and providing loans which do not exceed the cost of attendance (tuition, reasonable educational expenses and reasonable living expenses). You are eligible to apply for this loan if you are from a disadvantaged background as defined by the U.S. Department of Health and Human Services and are a citizen, national, or a lawful permanent resident of the United States or the District of Columbia, the Commonwealths of Puerto Rico or the Marianas Islands, the Virgin Islands, Guam, the American Samoa, the Trust Territory of the Pacific Islands, the Republic of Palau, the Republic of the Marshall Islands and the Federated State of Micronesia. Check to see if your school participates in the program.
- **Global Health Education Loan Program (GHELP).** A Global Health Education Loan can finance up to 100% of the cost of foreign medical school, as long as it is an eligible institution. GHELP helps cover your medical education with a complete package of student loans, including a federal Stafford loan, a federal Graduate PLUS loan, a private education loan, and a residency loan option for students who have graduated from medical school and have to relocate. GHELP is administered by Sallie Mae. You should contact them for information about loan rates and fees, the types of schools eligible, and payment options.

Grants and Scholarships Available to Medical Students

Some grants for medical students are more general in nature while others are more specific and are designed to attract certain students. When applying for a grant, make sure that you read the eligibility criteria. To ensure that you have every opportunity to receive available grants: (1) visit the community foundation website and register for the Online Grant Application System at www.thecommunityfoundation.org, and (2) visit the financial aid office at the medical school as soon as you arrive and inquire about every grant and scholarship available. Each school has its own list of funds that they award each year. The following are just some of the grants available to medical school students:

- **AMA Foundation Scholarships.** The American Medical Association has a list of financial aid resources available for medical students, information about medical education financing and student debt, and other resources intended to aid students in locating and securing financial aid. To look for funding, visit the AMA website.
- **RSNA Research Grant.** The Radiological Society of North America established this grant for students interested in radiology. The student is awarded $6,000 to participate in a 10-week research project in radiology, nuclear medicine, or oncology radiation. Preference is usually given to medical students who have research experience in medical imaging. Application is through the Online Grant Application System.
- **The Academic Research Enhancement Award (AREA).** NIH established the Academic Research Enhancement Award for students conducting research and attending a health professional school. To be eligible, a student must be enrolled in any academic health program including medicine, dentistry, osteopathy, nursing, pharmacy, optometry, allied health, public health, podiatry, veterinary medicine, nutrition, veterinary medicine, and chiropractic medicine.
- **Medical Research Fellows Program.** This program awards up to 20 fellowships annually to assist medical, dental, and veterinary students advance biomedical research from the laboratory into the treatment of disease. An 8-10-week summer program offers first or second year students who are attending schools in the United States the opportunity to do research in the laboratory of a Howard Hughes investigator, early career scientist, or a Howard Hughes Medical Institute professor.
- **Herbert W. Nickens Medical Student Scholarships.** This scholarship assists medical school candidates entering their third year of studies and who have demonstrated leadership in the needs of minorities in the United States. To be eligible, you must have exhibited an interest and commitment to health care in minority communities.
- **NIH Grants and Funding.** A number of funding opportunities are available for medical students through the National Institutes of Health. To search for NIH grants, visit their funding website at http://grants.nih.gov/grants/oer.htm.

To learn more about applying for grants, as well as a list of grants available, the following websites that will help you identify funding opportunities.

1. **Fastweb**: http://edu.fastweb.com/v/o_registration/flow/step1
2. **Scholarships.com** at https://www.scholarships.com
3. **Student Scholarship Search** at http://www.studentscholarshipsearch.com

Need-Based Financial Aid

Many schools place a high priority on need-based financial assistance for its student's in the form of grants, low-interest loans, or a combination of both. At one school, for example, more than 80 percent of the total student enrollment received financial assistance from a source other than parents. Some schools would rather offer grants to needy students to minimize the student's loan debt following graduation.

Need-based financial aid is offered to both state resident and non-resident students and it can vary from school to school. Typically, a medical school will also have endowed scholarships, and students are selected based on criteria established by the donor of the scholarship. You should check the individual school for any specific rules or deadlines, etc.

Merit Awards

Merit awards are based on academic excellence and may have certain criteria attached to them such as minority status, extracurricular activities, or service and/or leadership in the community. Each medical school has a limited number of these merit scholarships, but they can be substantial (full tuition for four years as an example). Annual renewal of awards is often contingent upon satisfactory academic progress, which is defined by the medical school. In some cases, merit awards are only given to residents of the state in which the medical school is located. Others are open to any applicant. You need to check with the financial aid officer to see if you qualify.

Armed Forces Health Professions Scholarship Program (HPSP)

One of the most comprehensive scholarships available in the health care field, the Armed Forces Health Professions Scholarship Program awards qualifying students full tuition for any accredited medical, dental, veterinary, psychology, or optometry program, plus a monthly stipend of nearly $3,000. Also covered is cost of books, equipment, and academic fees. Qualifying medical and dental students are also eligible to receive sign-on bonuses. After graduation, you will enter active duty in your specialty and advance in rank to captain. With every promotion, your salary would increase. Additionally, you receive a monthly non-taxable allowance for food and housing. To qualify for HPSP, you must:

1. Be a U.S. citizen with a baccalaureate degree from an accredited school.
2. Be enrolled in (or have a letter or acceptance from) an accredited graduate program in the U.S. or Puerto Rico (varies by specialty).
3. Maintain full-time student status during the length of the program.
4. Qualify as a commissioned officer.

Your active duty service obligation to the U.S. Army is one year of service for every year you receive the scholarship. Your minimum obligation depends on your health care field, and there is an additional obligation for residency and fellowship training.

Medical School Stafford Loan

Formerly known as the Guaranteed Student Loan or GSL, the Stafford Loan, administered by Sallie Mae, is the most common type of financial assistance for medical students. The following is an overview of the requirements and regulations:

- **Who is eligible?** Medical students who are U.S. citizens, legal permanent residents, or eligible non-citizens who have been accepted at a U.S. medical school. Students cannot have defaulted on other federal student loans in the past and must attend school at least half time to qualify.
- **How much can I borrow?** Medical students can borrow up to $20,500 a year in Stafford loans, and up to $138,500 total for their studies. Students in certain specialties have higher maximums and can borrow up to $47,167 a year and up to $224,000 in total through the Stafford program.
- **What is the interest rate?** Stafford loan interest rates are determined annually using the interest rate on the 10-year Treasury note. The most recent rate for graduate students is the interest rate of the note plus 3.6 percent, with a cap of 9.5 percent. Because rates are market-based, they fluctuate from year to year, but once the loan is issued, the rate is locked in. All Stafford loans for graduate students are unsubsidized, which means that interest will accumulate while students are in school.
- **How do I apply?** Applicants must fill out a FAFSA. For Stafford loans, students do not need to demonstrate financial need. Students are not eligible for a Stafford loan if they are part-time students or if they have defaulted on other college loans. Students who have defaulted on a mortgage, car, credit card or medical bills are still eligible to apply.
- **How do I repay the loan?** The first payment is due six months after you have graduated or after you have dropped out. And unlike a mortgage or credit card debt, which can be forgiven if you file for bankruptcy, a Stafford loan must be repaid.

Financial Aid for Disadvantaged Health Professions Students (FADHPS)

Applicants for FADHPS, which was established in 1987, are selected by the medical school based on financial need and federal guidelines. The main criteria is that the student be from a disadvantaged background or from a low-income family. The student's financial resources must not exceed the lesser of $5,000 or one half of the cost of the medical education.

Following graduation, the student must enter a residency program in a primary healthcare field like family practice, general internal medicine, general pediatrics, or preventive medicine/public health not later than four years after completing his or her medical education, then practice in primary care for five years after completion of the residency. Students who fail to meet academic standards or graduates who fail to comply with the primary care requirements will be liable to the federal government for the amount of the award plus any interest.

National Health Services Corps Scholarship Program (NHSC)

NHSC scholarships provide money for tuition, fees, books, supplies, equipment, and a monthly stipend for up to four years of medical school. The following criteria are used to determine eligibility:

1. Be a U.S. citizen attending a U.S. medical school.
2. Preference is given to students interested in primary health care specialties.
3. Preference is given to prior NHSC recipients and disadvantaged backgrounds.

Applicants who are considered will be interviewed and, if they accept, agree to serve one year of full-time clinical primary health care services for each year of support. The minimum obligation is two years. For more information, students can get applications from a financial aid officer or by contacting the NHSC Scholarship Program at 1-800-221-9393.

Primary Care Loan (PCL)

The Primary Care Loan program provides long-term, low interest rate loans to full-time, financially needy students to pursue a degree in allopathic or osteopathic medicine. Loans to third- and fourth-year students may be increased to repay outstanding balances on other loans taken out while in attendance at that school. Medical students receiving a Primary Care Loan must agree to (1) enter and complete residency training in primary care within four years after graduation and (2) practice in primary care for the life of the loan. You are eligible to apply for this loan at a school that participates in the Primary Care Loan program if you are:

- A citizen, national, or a lawful permanent resident of the United States or the District of Columbia, the Commonwealths of Puerto Rico or the Marianas Islands, the Virgin Islands, Guam, the American Samoa, the Trust Territory of the Pacific Islands, the Republic of Palau, the Republic of the Marshall Islands and the Federated State of Micronesia.
- Enrolled as a full-time student at an accredited, participating school in a degree program leading to a Doctor of Medicine or doctor of osteopathy.
- Able to demonstrate financial need and provide financial information about your parents (independent students do not have to provide parental financial information, but must be at least 24 years of age and must provide documentation showing that you have been independent for a minimum of 3 years).
- Not in default on any federal loan and owe no federal grant refund.
- In good academic standing.
- Registered with Selective Service if required by law.

Loan Specifics

The PCL interest rate is 5 percent and begins to accrue following a one-year grace period after you cease to be a full-time student. The loan also offers deferment of principal and interest not found in other loan programs. The financial aid office at the participating school where you are enrolled will determine how much you can borrow based on your eligibility, the amount of PCL funds available at your institution and other criteria. The maximum award for first- and second- year students is cost of attendance (including tuition, educational expenses, and reasonable living expenses). Amounts beyond this may be awarded to third- and fourth-year students.

Primary Care Requirements

New recipients of the Primary Care Loan must enter into a residency training program in family medicine, internal medicine, pediatrics, combined medicine/pediatrics, preventive medicine, or osteopathic general practice; must complete the residency program within 4 years of graduation; and must practice primary care for either 10 years (including the years spent in residency training) or through the date on which the loan is repaid in full, whichever occurs first. Recipients of loans made prior to March 23, 2010 are required to practice in primary health care until the loan is paid in full.

Primary Care: Acceptable Specialties

Clinical Preventive Medicine, Occupational Medicine, Public Health, Public Policy Fellowship, Geriatrics, Adolescent Medicine, Adolescent Pediatrics, Sports Medicine

Non-Primary Care: Unacceptable Specialties

Cardiology, Gastroenterology, Obstetrics/Gynecology, Surgery, Dermatology, Radiology, Rehabilitation Medicine, Psychiatry, Emergency Medicine

The primary health care service obligation may be waived if you terminate studies before graduating and do not later resume studies or suspended for the period you are not enrolled because you have terminated studies before graduating; your obligation is resumed when you return to medical school to complete your studies. Should you fail to fulfill the service obligation, the outstanding loan balance will be computed annually at an interest rate of 2 percent greater than the rate you would pay if compliant.

For recipients of loans made prior to March 23, 2010 who fail to fulfill the service obligation, the outstanding loan balance will be computed annually at an interest rate of 18 percent from the date of noncompliance. If you are not committed to the practice of primary health care, you should not accept a Primary Care Loan.

You may obtain additional certification in primary health care while fulfilling your service obligation if you complete your primary health care residency program within four years after graduation. For example, if your primary care residency is completed in 3 years after graduation, you may obtain certification in an area of training to enhance your primary health care practice (i.e., geriatrics) at any time, and it will be considered an acceptable activity for fulfillment of your service obligation.

Repayment

Repayment begins following a 12-month grace period after you cease to be a full-time student. Interest at 5 percent is computed on the unpaid principal balance and begins to accrue upon expiration of your grace period unless you are eligible to defer payment. Loans are repayable over a period of not less than 10 years or more than 25 years, at the discretion of the institution. Repayment of the Primary Care Loan may be deferred for:

- Up to 4 years in an eligible primary health care residency program.

- Up to 3 years as a volunteer under the Peace Corps Act practicing in an eligible primary health care activity.
- Up to 3 years as a member of a uniformed service. To be eligible, you must be on sustained full-time active duty practicing in an eligible primary health care activity in the Army, Navy, Air Force, Marine Corps, Coast Guard, National Oceanic and Atmospheric Administration Corps or the U.S. Public Health Service Commissioned Corps.

The Primary Care Loan is not eligible for consolidation because of the service obligation. In the unfortunate event of the borrower's death or total disability, the obligation to repay the loan will be canceled upon receipt of the required documentation.

Other Types of Financial Assistance

Besides scholarships, grants, merit awards, and federal loans based on financial need and/or minority/disadvantaged status, other types of financial aid are available for medical students. No candidate will ever be turned away because he or she cannot afford medical school. The school's financial aid officer should have a list of everything the school offers, as well as information about certain types of financial aid not offered directly through the financial aid office. Some other types of financial aid you may want to get information about are:

Medical Student Research Scholarships: Most medical schools have research programs conducted by faculty and staff. Not only do students get valuable experience and a scholarship for participating in research, they often get credit toward their basic sciences.

Funds for In-State Students: Residents should fill out appropriate forms for "state-sponsored" scholarships immediately after being accepted for admission. Sometimes there is a separate financial aid form other than the one completed for other types of financial aid. And since these are limited and given away quickly, you need to get the forms in well before the deadline.

Funds for Combined Degree Programs: Highly qualified and motivated students wanting to spend 6 to 7 years studying for a combined M.D./Ph.D. degree may qualify for funding available specifically for them. Typically, funding for a combined M.D./Ph.D. candidate will be available for up to six years, though the six years need not be consecutive. Other combined degree programs that qualify are: M.D./J.D. degree, M.D./M.P.H. degree, and M.D./M.B.A. degree.

Private Endowments: Though not common, there are some corporations that make funds available directly to students. The majority, though, distribute funds to medical schools, which then award these funds to the medical students. If there are some scholarships or grants available through these channels, the financial aid officer will have either the information or the applications.

CHAPTER 12

HEALTH CAREERS FOR THE 21ST CENTURY

Despite their best efforts, and no matter how many times they try, some students simply will not get admitted to medical school. If you're one of those students, there are many other outstanding careers in healthcare. Keep in mind, though, that some professional programs such as physician assistant or physical therapy may be just as difficult to get into. Physician assistant programs, for example, require experience in the medical field to even be considered. So do your homework and know what's required to qualify for one of these programs.

If you're set on making healthcare your career, and want to spend time with patients, consider alternate fields such as nurse practitioner, chiropractic, physical therapy, or podiatry. All these fields involve the science and art of diagnosis, treatment, and healing, but they differ in the methods of treatment they use and in their areas of specialty. Some of the greatest increases in employment over the next few decades will be in various fields of healthcare; so if going to medical school is not in your future, there's no reason why you still can't have a rewarding career.

Top 10 Healthcare Careers of the Future

Over the next few decades, jobs in healthcare will grow more rapidly than just about any other field. With new healthcare laws and regulations, the entire landscape of healthcare is changing, and, in many cases, physicians will not be at the front lines of patient care. That responsibility will go to healthcare providers like physician assistants and nurse practitioners. The following, according to leading experts in the field, are the top healthcare careers of the future, some of them projected to grow by as much as 40% over the next decade. Descriptions are based on the Bureau of Labor Statistics and the U.S. Government's Occupational Outlook Handbook.

1. Physician Assistant

With rapid growth in the health care field, more and more hospitals and HMOs are depending on physician assistants to help provide quality health care. Most of the PAs work in primary care, especially in underserved rural areas and inner cities where traditionally there are few physicians. More recently, however, PAs have become increasingly involved in every medical specialty and subspecialty. And according to the U.S. Department of Labor, there will be nearly a 60 percent increase in the number of PA positions by end of the decade, making this field one of the fastest growing in the health care industry. A physician assistant's duties include:

- Reviewing patients' medical histories.
- Conducting physical exams to check patients' health.
- Ordering and interpreting diagnostic tests, such as x rays or blood tests.
- Making diagnoses concerning a patient's injury or illness.
- Giving treatment, such as setting broken bones and immunizing patients.
- Educating and counseling patients and their families.
- Prescribing medicine when needed.
- Recording a patient's progress.
- Researching the latest treatments to ensure the quality of patient care.
- Conducting or participate in outreach programs, talking to groups about managing diseases and promoting wellness.

Currently there are 309 accredited U.S. programs offering the PA. Students use a centralized application service, much like the AMCAS for medical school, called the Central Application Service for Physician Assistants or CASPA. Requirements vary from school to school, but most require a 4-year degree and clinical experience. The physician assistant program at some PA schools requires that applicants have six months of full-time employment or 1000 hours of hands-on health care experience. For more specific admission requirements, look at each individual program's catalogue.

The physician assistant curriculum typically includes both classroom and clinical instruction. The first year is spent studying medical sciences such as anatomy, physiology, pharmacology, laboratory medicine, emergency medical training, and physical assessment. The second year is spent in clinical settings, where students participate in patient care and serve in clerkships. Students wanting more information on individual programs should contact the school directly. For information and a list of Physician Assistant programs throughout the United States, visit the American Academy of Physician Assistants at www.aapa.org.

2. Registered Nurse

Registered nurses (RNs) provide and coordinate patient care, educate patients and the public about various health conditions, and provide advice and emotional support to patients and their family members. Duties include:

- Recording patients' medical histories and symptoms.
- Administering patients' medicines and treatments.
- Setting up plans for patients' care or contributing to existing plans.
- Observing patients and recording observations.
- Consulting with doctors and other healthcare professionals.

- Operating and monitoring medical equipment.
- Helping perform diagnostic tests and analyzing results.
- Teaching patients and their families how to manage illnesses or injuries.
- Explaining what to do at home after treatment.

Most registered nurses work as part of a team with physicians and other healthcare specialists. Some registered nurses oversee licensed practical nurses, nursing assistants, and home health aides. Registered nurses' duties and titles often depend on where they work and the patients they work with. Some registered nurses combine one or more specific areas. For example, a pediatric oncology nurse works with children and teens that have cancer. Many possibilities for working with specific patient groups exist. The following list includes just a few examples:

Addiction nurses: care for patients who need help to overcome addictions to alcohol, drugs, tobacco, and other substances.

Cardiovascular nurses: care for patients with heart disease and people who have had heart surgery.

Critical care nurses: work in intensive care units in hospitals, providing care to patients with serious, complex, and acute illnesses and injuries that need close monitoring and treatment.

Genetics nurses: provide screening, counseling, and treatment of patients with genetic disorders, such as cystic fibrosis.

Neonatology nurses: take care of newborn babies.

Nephrology nurses: care for patients who have kidney-related health issues stemming from diabetes, high blood pressure, substance abuse, or other causes.

Rehabilitation nurses: care for patients with temporary or permanent disabilities.

Some nurses have jobs in which they do not work directly with patients, but they must still have an active registered nurse license. For example, they may work as nurse educators, healthcare consultants, public policy advisors, researchers, hospital administrators, salespeople for pharmaceutical and medical supply companies, or as medical writers and editors.

Registered nurses usually take one of three education paths: A Bachelor of Science degree in nursing (BSN), an associate degree in nursing (ADN), or a diploma from an approved nursing program. Registered nurses also must be licensed. To learn more about careers in nursing, visit the American Nurses Association at http://nursingworld.org.

3. Nurse Practitioner

Nurse practitioners or NPs serve as primary and specialty care providers, providing advanced nursing services to patients and their families. NPs assess patients, determine the best way to improve or manage a patient's health, and discuss ways to integrate health promotion strategies into a patient's life. They typically care for a certain population of people. For instance, NPs may work in adult and geriatric health, pediatric health, or psychiatric and mental health. Although the scope of their duties varies by state, many nurse practitioners work independently, prescribe medications, and order laboratory tests. All nurse practitioners consult with physicians and other health professionals when needed.

NPs who work with patients typically perform many of the same duties as registered nurses, gathering information about a patient's condition and taking action to treat or manage the patient's health. However, PNs are also trained to perform additional functions because they are often the first healthcare provider a patient will see. Because of the growing demand for non-physician healthcare providers, their principle duties might include:

- Setting up plans for patients' care.
- Performing physical exams.
- Diagnosing various health problems.
- Performing and ordering diagnostic tests and analyzing results.
- Giving patients medicines and treatments.
- Operating and monitoring medical equipment.
- Provide counseling and teaching patients and their families how to stay healthy or manage their illnesses or injuries.
- Conducting research.
- Participating in community outreach programs.

The requirements for a nurse practitioner are a bachelor's degree in nursing and two additional years in a nurse practitioner training program leading to a master's degree in nursing. To learn more about a career as a nurse practitioner, visit the American Association of Nurse Practitioners at http://www.aanp.org.

4. Physical Therapist

Physical therapists, sometimes called PTs, help injured or ill people improve their movement and manage their pain. These therapists are often an important part of rehabilitation and the treatment of patients with chronic conditions or injuries. Their duties include:

- Reviewing patients' medical history and referrals or notes from doctors or surgeons.
- Diagnosing patients' dysfunctional movements by observing them stand or walk and by listening to their concerns, among other methods.
- Setting up a plan of care for patients and outlining the patient's goals and the expected outcome of the plan.
- Using exercises, stretching maneuvers, hands-on therapy, and equipment to ease patients' pain, help them increase their mobility, prevent further pain or injury, and facilitate health and wellness.
- Evaluating a patient's progress, modifying a plan of care, and trying new treatments.

- Educating patients and their families about what to expect from and how best to cope with the recovery process.

Physical therapists provide care to people of all ages who have functional problems resulting from back and neck injuries, sprains, strains, and fractures, arthritis, amputations, neurological disorders, such as stroke or cerebral palsy, injuries related to work and sports, and other conditions. They're trained to use a variety of techniques—sometimes called modalities—to care for their patients. These techniques include applying heat and cold and using assistive devices such as crutches, wheelchairs, walkers, and adhesive electrodes that apply electric stimulation to treat injuries and pain.

Some physical therapists specialize in one type of care, such as orthopedics or geriatrics. They often work as part of a healthcare team, overseeing the work of physical therapist assistants and aides and consulting with physicians and surgeons and other specialists. To become a physical therapist, a person must obtain a graduate degree. College programs in physical therapy are typically a combination of coursework and clinical rotations in hospitals or other healthcare settings. Additionally, states require individuals to be licensed to legally work in this career. To learn more about a physical therapy, visit the American Physical Therapy Association at http://www.apta.org.

5. Occupational Therapist

Occupational therapists treat injured, ill, or disabled patients through the therapeutic use of everyday activities. They help these patients develop, recover, and improve the skills needed for daily living and working. Their duties include:

- Observing patients doing tasks and reviewing their medical history.
- Evaluating a patient's condition and needs.
- Developing a treatment plan, activities, and goals for patients.
- Helping people with various disabilities perform different tasks.
- Prescribing exercises that can help relieve pain for people with chronic conditions.
- Evaluating a patient's home or workplace and identifying potential improvements.
- Educating a patient's family and employer about how to accommodate and care for the patient.
- Recommending special equipment, such as wheelchairs and eating aids, and instructing patients on how to use that equipment.
- Assessing and recording patients' activities and progress for patient evaluations, for billing, and for reporting to physicians and other healthcare providers.

Some occupational therapists work with children in educational settings. They evaluate disabled children's abilities, modify classroom equipment to accommodate children with certain disabilities, and help children participate in school activities. Some therapists who work with the elderly help their patients lead more independent and active lives. They assess patients' abilities and environment and make recommendations. For example, therapists may identify potential fall hazards in a patient's home and recommend their removal. In some cases, occupational therapists help create functional work environments. They evaluate the workspace, plan work activities, and meet with the patient's employer to collaborate on changes to the patient's work environment or schedule.

Some occupational therapists, such as those employed in hospitals, work as part of a healthcare team along with doctors, registered nurses, and other types of therapists. They may work with patients with chronic conditions, such as diabetes, or help rehabilitate a patient recovering from a hip replacement surgery. Occupational therapists also oversee the work of occupational therapy assistants and aides. To become an occupational therapist, you must have a master's degree and be licensed by the state in which you practice. To learn more about the requirements and a career in occupational therapy, visit the American Occupational Therapy Association website at http://www.aota.org.

6. Radiologic Technologist

Radiologic technologists perform diagnostic imaging examinations, such as x rays, on patients. Their duties include:

- Adjusting and maintaining imaging equipment.
- Precisely following orders from physicians on what areas of the body to image.
- Preparing patients for procedures, including taking a medical history and answering questions about the procedure.
- Operating the computerized equipment to take the images.
- Working with physicians to evaluate the images and to determine whether additional images need to be taken.
- Keeping detailed patient records.

Healthcare professionals use many types of equipment to diagnose patients. Radiologic technologists specialize in x-ray and computed tomography (CT) imaging. Some radiologic technologists prepare a mixture for the patient to drink that allows soft tissue to be viewed on the images that the radiologist reviews. Radiologic technologists might also specialize in mammography, the use of low-dose x-ray systems to produce images of the breast. Technologists may be certified in multiple specialties.

To enter a training program for radiologic technology, applicants usually require at least a high school diploma or a GED. Prospective radiologic technologists receive training at a program accredited by the Joint Review Committee on Education in Radiologic Technology, which can be at a trade school, a community college, or a traditional university. These programs last between one and four years and result in a certificate of completion or an associate or bachelor's degree. To learn more about a career in radiologic technology, visit the American Society of Radiologic Technologists at http://www.asrt.org.

7. Pharmacist

Pharmacists dispense prescription medications to patients and offer expertise in the safe use of prescriptions. They also may provide advice on how to lead a healthy lifestyle, conduct health and wellness screenings, provide immunizations, and oversee the medications given to patients. Duties include:

- Filling prescriptions and verifying instructions from physicians on the proper amounts of medication to give to patients.
- Checking whether the prescription will interact negatively with other drugs that a patient is taking or any medical conditions the patient has.
- Instructing patients on how and when to take a prescribed medicine and informing them about potential side effects.
- Advising patients about general health topics such as diet, exercise, managing stress, and on other issues such as what equipment or supplies would be best to treat a health problem.
- Giving flu shots and, in most states, other vaccinations.
- Completing insurance forms and working with insurance companies to ensure that patients get the medicines they need.
- Overseeing the work of pharmacy technicians and pharmacists in training (interns).
- Keeping records and doing other administrative tasks.
- Teaching other healthcare practitioners about proper medication therapies for patients.

Some pharmacists who own their pharmacy or manage a chain pharmacy spend time on business activities, such as inventory management. Pharmacists must also take continuing education courses throughout their career to keep up with the latest advances in pharmacological science. Some pharmacists create customized medications by mixing ingredients themselves, a process known as compounding. The following are examples of types of pharmacists:

Community pharmacists: work in retail stores such as chain drug stores or independently owned pharmacies. They dispense medications to patients and answer any questions that patients may have about prescriptions, over-the-counter medications, or any health concerns that the patient may have. They may also provide some primary care services such as giving flu shots.

Clinical pharmacists: work in hospitals, clinics, and other healthcare settings. They spend little time dispensing prescriptions. Instead, they are involved in direct patient care. Clinical pharmacists may go on rounds in a hospital with a physician or healthcare team. They recommend medications to give to patients and oversee the dosage and timing of the delivery of those medications. They may also conduct some medical tests and offer advice to patients. For example, pharmacists working in a diabetes clinic may counsel patients on how and when to take medications, suggest healthy food choices, and monitor patients' blood sugar.

Consultant pharmacists: advise healthcare facilities or insurance providers on patient medication use or improving pharmacy services. They also may give advice directly to patients, such as helping seniors manage their prescriptions.

Pharmaceutical industry pharmacists: work in areas such as marketing, sales, or research and development. They may design or conduct clinical drug trials and help to develop new drugs. They also may help to establish safety regulations and ensure quality control for drugs.

Pharmacists must have a Doctor of Pharmacy (Pharm.D.) degree from a pharmacy program accredited by the Accreditation Council for Pharmacy Education. They also must be licensed, which requires passing licensure and law exams. For more information, visit the American Pharmacists Association at http://www.pharmacist.com.

8. Healthcare Administrative Manager

Healthcare administrators plan, direct, and coordinate medical and health services. They might manage an entire facility or specialize in managing a specific clinical area or department or manage a medical practice for a group of physicians. Medical and health services managers must be able to adapt to changes in healthcare laws, regulations, and technology. Duties include:

- Working to improve efficiency and quality in delivering healthcare services.
- Keeping up to date on new laws and regulations so that the facility in which they work complies with them.
- Supervising assistant administrators in facilities that are large enough to need them.
- Managing the finances of the facility, such as patient fees and billing.
- Representing the facility at investor meetings or on governing boards.
- Keeping and organizing records of the facility's services, such as the number of inpatient beds used.
- Facilitating conferences and meetings for staff.
- Communicating with members of the medical staff and department heads.

In group medical practices, managers work closely with physicians and surgeons, registered nurses, medical and clinical laboratory technologists and technicians and other healthcare workers. Medical and health services managers' titles depend on the facility or area of expertise in which they work. The following are some examples of types of medical and health services managers:

Nursing home administrators: manage staff, admissions, finances, and care of the building, as well as care of the residents in nursing homes. All states require them to be licensed; licensing requirements vary by state.

Clinical managers: oversee a specific department, such as nursing, surgery, or physical therapy, and have responsibilities based on that specialty. Clinical managers set and carry out policies, goals, and procedures for their departments; evaluate the quality of the staff's work; and develop reports and budgets.

Health information managers: responsible for the maintenance and security of all patient records. They must stay up to date with evolving information technology and current or proposed laws about health information systems. Health information managers must ensure that databases are complete, accurate, and accessible only to authorized personnel.

Assistant administrators: work under the top administrator in larger facilities and often handle daily decisions. Assistants might direct activities in clinical areas, such as nursing, surgery, therapy, medical records, or health information. Most healthcare managers have at least a bachelor's degree before entering the field. However, a master's degree is common. Requirements vary by facility. To learn more about a career in healthcare management visit the American Association of Healthcare Administrative Management at http://www.aaham.org.

9. Healthcare Information Technician

Medical records and health information technicians organize and manage health information data by ensuring its quality, accuracy, accessibility, and security in both paper and electronic systems. They use various classification systems to code and categorize patient information for insurance reimbursement purposes, for databases and registries, and to maintain patients' medical and treatment histories. Duties include:

- Reviewing patient records for completeness, accuracy, and appropriateness of data.
- Organizing and maintaining data for clinical databases and registries.
- Tracking patient outcomes for quality assessment.
- Using classification software to assign codes for reimbursement and data analysis.
- Electronically recording data for collection, storage, analysis, retrieval, and reporting.
- Protecting patients' health information for confidentiality, authorized access for treatment, and data security.

All health information technicians document patients' health information, including their medical history, symptoms, examination and test results, treatments, and other information about healthcare services that are provided to patients. Their duties vary with the size of the facility in which they work. Although health information technicians do not provide direct patient care, they work regularly with registered nurses and other healthcare professionals. They meet with these workers to clarify diagnoses or to get additional information to make sure that records are complete and accurate.

The increasing use of electronic health records (EHRs) will continue to change the job responsibilities of health information technicians. Federal legislation provides incentives for physicians' offices and hospitals to implement EHR systems into their practice. This will lead to continued adoption of this software in these facilities. Technicians will need to be familiar with, or be able to learn, EHR computer software, follow EHR security and privacy practices, and analyze electronic data to improve healthcare information as more healthcare providers and hospitals adopt EHR systems.

Medical laboratory technologists typically need a bachelor's degree. Technicians usually need an associate degree or a postsecondary certificate. Some states require technologists and technicians to be licensed. To learn more about a career in healthcare information technology, visit Health Information Technology at http://www.aha.org/advocacy-issues/hit /index.shtml.

10. Medical Laboratory Technologist or Technician

Medical laboratory technologists and medical laboratory technicians collect samples and perform tests to analyze body fluids, tissue, and other substances. Medical laboratory technologists perform complex medical laboratory tests; medical laboratory technicians perform routine medical laboratory tests. Duties include:

- Analyzing body fluids, such as blood, urine, and tissue samples, and recording normal or abnormal findings.
- Studying blood samples for use in transfusions by identifying the number of cells, the cell morphology or the blood group, blood type, and compatibility with other blood types.
- Operating sophisticated laboratory equipment such as microscopes and cell counters.
- Using automated equipment and computerized instruments capable of performing several tests at the same time.
- Logging data from medical tests and entering results into a patient's medical record.
- Discussing results and findings of laboratory tests and procedures with physicians.
- Supervising or training medical laboratory technicians.

Both technicians and technologists perform tests and procedures that physicians and surgeons or other healthcare personnel order. However, technologists perform more complex tests and laboratory procedures than technicians do. For example, technologists may prepare specimens and perform manual tests that are based on detailed instructions, whereas technicians perform routine tests that may be more automated. Medical laboratory technicians usually work under the general supervision of medical laboratory technologists or laboratory managers.

Technologists in small laboratories perform many types of tests; in large laboratories, they generally specialize. The following are examples of specialized medical laboratory technologists:

Blood bank technologists or immunohematology technologists: collect blood, classify it by type, and prepare blood and its components for transfusions.

Clinical chemistry technologists: prepare specimens and analyze the chemical and hormonal contents of body fluids.

Cytotechnologists: prepare slides of body cells and examine these cells with a microscope for abnormalities that may signal the beginning of a cancerous growth.

Immunology technologists: examine elements of the human immune system and its response to foreign bodies.

Microbiology technologists: examine and identify bacteria and other microorganisms.

Molecular biology technologists: perform complex protein and nucleic acid tests on cell samples.

Like technologists, medical laboratory technicians may work in several areas of the laboratory or specialize in one area. Technologists and technicians often specialize after they've worked in a particular area for a long time or have received advanced education or training in that area. Medical laboratory technologists typically need a bachelor's degree. Technicians usually need an associate degree or a postsecondary certificate. Some states require technologists and technicians to be licensed. To learn more about medical technology, visit American Medical Technologists at http://american medtech.org.

Other Health-Related Careers

There are many careers in healthcare, and with the population growing and aging, the need for healthcare workers in all areas will also grow. The following are descriptions of other health-related careers that would provide a challenging and rewarding lifetime career.

Audiology: Audiologists diagnose and treat a patient's hearing and balance problems, using advanced technology and procedures. Duties include:

- Examining patients who have hearing, balance, or related ear problems.
- Assessing the results of the examination and diagnose problems.
- Determining and administering treatment.
- Administering relief procedures for various forms of vertigo.
- Fitting and dispensing hearing aids.
- Counseling patients and their families on ways to listen and communicate, such as by lip reading or through American Sign Language.

Audiologists use audiometers, computers, and other devices to test patients' hearing ability and balance, to determine the extent of hearing damage, and to identify the underlying cause. Treatment may include cleaning wax out of ear canals, fitting and checking hearing aids, or fitting the patient with cochlear implants to improve hearing. Audiologists can also help patients suffering from vertigo or dizziness by providing them with exercises involving head movement or positioning that might relieve symptoms. Some audiologists specialize in working with the elderly or with children. Others design products to help protect the hearing of workers on the job. Audiologists need a doctoral degree and must be licensed in all states. To learn more, visit http://www.asha.org.

Chiropractic: Chiropractors care for patients with health problems of the neuromusculoskeletal system, which includes nerves, bones, muscles, ligaments, and tendons. They use spinal adjustments, manipulation, and other techniques to manage patients' health concerns, such as back and neck pain. Duties include:

- Assessing a patient's medical condition by reviewing their medical history, listening to the patient's concerns, and performing a physical examination.
- Analyzing the patient's posture, spine, and reflexes.
- Conducting tests, including evaluating a patient's posture and taking x rays.

- Identifying health problems.
- Providing neuromusculoskeletal therapy, which involves adjusting a patient's spinal column and other joints by hand.
- Giving additional treatments such as applying heat or cold to a patient's injured areas.
- Advising patients on health and lifestyle issues, such as exercise, nutrition, and sleep habits.
- Referring patients to other health care professionals, if needed.

Chiropractors focus on patients' overall health. They work on the belief that misalignments of the spinal joints interfere with a person's neuromuscular system and can result in lower resistance to disease, as well as other conditions of poor health. Some chiropractors use procedures such as massage therapy, rehabilitative exercise, and ultrasound in addition to spinal adjustments and manipulation. They also may apply supports, such as braces or shoe inserts, to treat patients and relieve pain. In addition to operating a general chiropractic practice, some chiropractors concentrate in areas such as sports, neurology, orthopedics, pediatrics, or nutrition, among others.

Chiropractors must earn a Doctor of Chiropractic (D.C.) degree and a state license. Doctor of Chiropractic programs typically take 4 years to complete and require at least 3 years of undergraduate college education for admission. For more information about chiropractic and a list of U.S. chiropractic colleges, visit the Council on Chiropractic Education at www.cce-usa.org.

Dental Hygiene: Dental hygienists clean teeth, examine patients for signs of oral diseases such as gingivitis, and provide other preventative dental care. They also educate patients on ways to improve and maintain good oral health. Duties include:

- Removing tartar, stains, and plaque from teeth.
- Applying sealants and fluorides to help protect teeth.
- Taking and developing dental x-rays.
- Keeping track of patient care and treatment plans.
- Teaching about oral hygiene techniques, such as how to brush and floss correctly.

Dental hygienists use many types of tools to do their job. They clean and polish teeth with hand, power, and ultrasonic tools. In some cases, they remove stains with an air-polishing device, which sprays a combination of air, water, and baking soda. They polish teeth with a powered tool that works like an automatic toothbrush. Hygienists use x-ray machines to take pictures to check for tooth or jaw problems. Some states allow hygienists to place and carve filling materials, temporary fillings, and periodontal dressings.

Dental hygienists typically need an associate degree in dental hygiene. All states require dental hygienists to be licensed. To learn more about dental hygienists, visit http://www.adha.org.

Dentistry: Dentists diagnose and treat problems with a patient's teeth, gums, and related parts of the mouth. They provide advice and instruction on taking care of teeth and gums and on diet choices that affect oral health. Duties include:

- Removing decay from teeth and fill cavities.
- Repairing cracked or fractured teeth and remove teeth.
- Straightening teeth to correct bite issues.
- Placing sealants or whitening agents on teeth.
- Writing prescriptions for antibiotics or other medications.
- Examining x-rays of teeth, gums, the jaw, and nearby areas for problems.
- Making models and measurements for dental appliances, such as dentures, to fit patients.
- Teaching patients about diet, flossing, use of fluoride and other aspects of dental care.

Dentists use a variety of equipment, including x-ray machines, drills, mouth mirrors, probes, forceps, brushes, and scalpels. They also use lasers, digital scanners, and other computer technologies. Most dentists are general practitioners and handle a variety of dental needs. Other dentists practice in one of nine specialty areas:

Dental public health specialists: promote good dental health and the prevention of dental diseases in specific communities.

Endodontists: perform root-canal therapy, by which they remove the nerves and blood supply from injured or infected teeth.

Oral and maxillofacial radiologists: diagnose diseases in the head and neck using imaging technologies.

Oral and maxillofacial surgeons: operate on the mouth, jaws, teeth, gums, neck, and head, including procedures such as surgically repairing a cleft lip and palate or removing impacted teeth.

Oral pathologists: diagnose conditions in the mouth, such as bumps or ulcers, and oral diseases, such as cancer.

Orthodontists: straighten teeth by applying pressure to the teeth with braces or other appliances.

Pediatric dentists: focus on dentistry for children and special-needs patients.

Periodontists: treat the gums and bone supporting the teeth.

Prosthodontists: replace missing teeth with permanent fixtures, such as crowns and bridges, or with removable fixtures such as dentures.

Dentists must be licensed in all states. To qualify for a license, applicants must graduate from an accredited dental school and pass written and practical exams. For additional information about requirements, the DAT, and a list of accredited dental schools, visit the American Dental Education Association at www.adea.org.

Dietetics/Nutrition: Dietitians and nutritionists are experts in food and nutrition. They advise people on what to eat in order to lead a healthy lifestyle or achieve a specific health-related goal. Duties include:

- Assessing patients' and clients' health needs and diet.
- Counseling patients on nutrition issues and healthy eating habits.
- Developing meal plans, taking both cost and clients' preferences into account.
- Evaluating the effects of meal plans and change the plans as needed.
- Promoting better nutrition by speaking to groups about diet, nutrition, and the relationship between good eating habits and preventing or managing specific diseases.
- Writing reports to document patient progress.

Dietitians and nutritionists evaluate the health of their clients. Based on their findings, dietitians and nutritionists advise clients on which foods to eat—and those foods to avoid—to improve their health. Some dietitians and nutritionists provide customized information for specific individuals. For example, a dietitian or nutritionist might teach a client with high blood pressure how to use less salt when preparing meals. Another might plan a diet with limited fat and sugar to help patients lose weight. Although many dietitians and nutritionists do similar tasks, there are several specialties within the occupations. The following are examples of types of dietitians and nutritionists:

Clinical dietitians and nutritionists: provide medical nutrition therapy. They work in hospitals, long-term care facilities, clinics, private practice, and other institutions. They create nutritional programs based on the health needs of patients or residents and counsel patients on how to lead a healthier lifestyle. Clinical dietitians and nutritionists may further specialize, such as working only with patients with kidney diseases or those with diabetes.

Community dietitians and nutritionists: develop programs and counsel the public on topics related to food and nutrition. They often work with specific groups of people, such as adolescents or the elderly. They work in public health clinics, government and nonprofit agencies, health maintenance organizations (HMOs), and other settings.

Management dietitians: plan meal programs. They work in food service settings such as cafeterias, hospitals, prisons, and schools. They may be responsible for buying food and for carrying out other business-related tasks such as budgeting. Management dietitians may oversee kitchen staff or other dietitians.

Most dietitians and nutritionists have a bachelor's degree and receive supervised training through an internship or as a part of their coursework. Many states require dietitians and nutritionists to be licensed. For more information, visit http://www.diet.com/store /facts/american-dietetic-association.

Exercise Physiology/Athletic Training: Exercise physiologists develop fitness and exercise programs that help patients recover from chronic diseases and improve cardiovascular function, body composition, and flexibility. Athletic trainers specialize in preventing, diagnosing, and treating muscle and bone injuries and illnesses.

Athletic trainers (ATs) typically do the following:

- Applying protective or injury-preventive devices such as tape, bandages, and braces.
- Recognizing and evaluating injuries.
- Providing first aid or emergency care.
- Developing and carrying out rehabilitation programs for injured athletes.
- Planning and implementing comprehensive programs to prevent injury and illness among athletes.
- Performing administrative tasks such as keeping records and writing reports on injuries and treatment programs.

Exercise physiologists (EPs) typically do the following:

- Analyzing a patient's medical history to determine the best possible exercise and fitness regimen.
- Performing fitness tests with medical equipment and analyzing patient data.
- Measuring body fat, blood pressure, oxygen use, and other patient health indicators.
- Developing exercise programs to improve patient health.
- Supervising clinical tests to ensure patient safety.

Athletic trainers work with people of all ages and all skill levels, from young children to soldiers and professional athletes, and are usually one of the first healthcare providers on the scene when injuries occur. They work under the direction of a licensed physician and with other healthcare providers, and often discuss specific injuries and treatment options or evaluate and treat patients as directed by a physician. Exercise physiologists work to improve overall patient health, and many of their patients suffer from health problems such as cardiovascular disease or are obese. Exercise physiologists provide health education and exercise plans to improve key health indicators. Some physiologists work closely with primary care physicians.

Athletic trainers and exercise physiologists should not be confused with fitness trainers and instructors, including personal trainers. Athletic trainers and exercise physiologists need at least a bachelor's degree. In most states, athletic trainers need a license or certification. For more information, visit http://www.nata. org and http://www.acsm-cepa.org.

Nurse Anesthetists, Nurse Midwives, and Nurse Practitioners: Nurse anesthetists, nurse midwives, and nurse practitioners, also referred to as advanced practice registered nurses (APRNs), coordinate patient care, and they may provide primary and specialty health care. The scope of practice varies from state to state. Duties include:

- Taking and recording patients' medical histories and symptoms and setting up plans for patients' care or contributing to existing plans.
- Performing physical exams.

- Observing patients and diagnosing various health problems.
- Performing and ordering diagnostic tests and analyze results.
- Giving patients medicines and treatments.
- Consulting with doctors and other healthcare professionals as needed.
- Operating and monitoring medical equipment.
- Providing counseling and teaching patients and their families how to stay healthy or manage their illnesses or injuries.

APRNs work independently or in collaboration with physicians. In most states, they can prescribe medications, order medical tests, and diagnose health problems. They may provide primary and preventative care and may specialize in care for certain groups of people, such as children, pregnant women, or patients with mental health disorders. APRNs who work with patients typically perform many of the same duties as registered nurses, gathering information about a patient's condition and taking action to treat or manage the patient's health. However, APRNs are also trained to perform many additional functions. The following are examples of types of APRNs:

Nurse anesthetists: provide anesthesia and related care before, during, and after surgical, therapeutic, diagnostic, and obstetrical procedures. They also provide pain management and some emergency services. Before a procedure begins, nurse anesthetists discuss with a patient any medications the patient is taking, as well as any allergies or illnesses the patient may have so that anesthesia can be safely administered. Nurse anesthetists then give a patient general anesthesia to put the patient to sleep or regional or local anesthesia to numb an area of the body. They remain with the patient throughout a procedure to monitor vital signs and adjust the anesthesia, as necessary.

Nurse midwives: provide care to women, including gynecological exams, family planning services, prenatal care, and attendance in labor and delivery. They may act as primary care providers for women and newborns. Many nurse midwives provide wellness care, educating their patients on how to lead healthy lives by discussing topics such as nutrition and disease prevention. Nurse midwives also provide care to their patients' partners for sexual or reproductive health issues.

Nurse practitioners (NPs): serve as primary and specialty care providers, providing advanced nursing services to patients and their families. NPs assess patients, determine the best way to improve or manage a patient's health, and discuss ways to integrate health promotion strategies into a patient's life. They typically care for a certain population of people. For instance, NPs may work in adult and geriatric health, pediatric health, or psychiatric and mental health. Although the scope of their duties varies some by state, many nurse practitioners work independently, prescribe medications and order laboratory tests. All nurse practitioners consult with physicians and other health professionals when needed.

Clinical nurse specialists (CNSs): provide direct patient care to a certain population of people, such as pediatric patients, within one of many nursing specialties, such as orthopedic nursing or oncology nursing. CNSs also provide indirect care by working with other nurses, healthcare teams, and various other staff to improve the quality of care that patients receive. They also work at the system or organizational level to improve the quality of nursing care throughout a facility related to their specialty. Those with a research doctorate may conduct research.

Nurse anesthetists, nurse midwives, and nurse practitioners must earn at least a master's degree in one of the specialty roles. APRNs must also be licensed registered nurses in their state and pass a national certification exam. To learn more about these professions, visit http://www.aana.com, http://www.midwife.org, and http://www.aanp.org.

Occupational Health & Safety: Occupational health and safety technicians collect data on the safety and health conditions of the workplace. Technicians work with occupational health and safety specialists in conducting tests and measuring hazards to help prevent harm to workers, property, the environment, and the general public. Duties include:

- Inspecting, testing, and evaluating workplace environments, equipment, and practices to ensure they follow safety standards and government regulations.
- Collecting samples of potentially toxic materials.
- Working with occupational health and safety specialists to fix hazardous and potentially hazardous conditions or equipment.
- Evaluating programs on workplace safety and health.
- Educating employers and workers about workplace safety.
- Demonstrating the correct use of safety equipment.
- Investigating incidents and accidents to identify what caused them and how they might be prevented in the future.

Technicians conduct tests and collect samples and measurements as part of workplace inspections. For example, they may collect and handle samples of dust, mold, gases, vapors, or other potentially hazardous materials. They test and identify work areas for potential health and safety hazards, examine and test machinery and equipment such as scaffolding and lifting devices to be sure that they meet appropriate safety regulations, and check that workers are using required protective gear, such as masks and hardhats. Technicians also check that hazardous materials are stored correctly. The following are examples of types of occupational health and safety technicians:

Health physics technicians: work in places that use radiation and radioactive material. Their goal is to protect people and the environment from hazardous radiation exposure.

Industrial or occupational hygiene technicians: examine the workplace for health hazards, such as exposure to lead, asbestos, pesticides, or contagious diseases.

Mine examiners: inspect mines for proper air flow and potential health hazards such as the buildup of methane or other harmful gases.

Occupational health and safety technicians typically enter the occupation through one of two paths. Some technicians learn through on-the-job training; others enter with postsecondary education such as an associate degree or certificate.

Optometry: Optometrists examine, diagnose, treat, and manage disorders of the visual system, eye diseases, and injuries. They prescribe eyeglasses or contact lenses as needed. Duties include:

- Performing vision tests and analyzing results.
- Diagnosing sight problems, such as nearsightedness or farsightedness and eye diseases, such as glaucoma.
- Prescribing eyeglasses, contact lenses, and medications.
- Providing treatments such as vision therapy or low-vision rehabilitation.
- Providing pre- and postoperative care to patients undergoing eye surgery.
- Evaluating patients for diseases such as diabetes and referring patients to other healthcare providers as needed.
- Promoting eye health by counseling patients.

Some optometrists spend much of their time providing specialized care, particularly if they are working in a group practice with other optometrists or physicians. For example, some optometrists mostly treat patients with only partial sight, a condition known as low vision. Others may focus on treating infants and children, working as postsecondary teachers, doing research in optometry colleges, or working as consultants in the eye care industry.

Optometrists should not be confused with ophthalmologists or opticians. Ophthalmologists are physicians who perform eye surgery and treat eye disease in addition to examining eyes and prescribing eyeglasses and contact lenses. Opticians fit and adjust eyeglasses. Optometrists must complete a Doctor of Optometry (O.D.) degree program and obtain a license to practice in a particular state. Doctor of Optometry programs take 4 years to complete, and most students have a bachelor's degree before entering an O.D. program. For additional information about optometry and a list of accredited optometry schools, visit the American Optometric Association at www.aoa.org.

Orthotics and Prosthetics: Orthotists and prosthetists, also called O&P professionals, design medical supportive devices and measure and fit patients for them. These devices include artificial limbs (arms, hands, legs, and feet), braces, and other medical or surgical devices. Duties include:

- Evaluating and interviewing patients to determine their needs.
- Measuring patients in order to design and fit medical devices.
- Designing orthopedic and prosthetic devices based on physicians' prescriptions.

- Taking a mold of the part of a patient's body that will be fitted with a brace or artificial limb.
- Selecting materials to be used for the orthotic or prosthetic device.
- Fitting, testing, and adjusting devices on patients.
- Instructing patients in how to use and care for their devices.
- Repairing or updating prosthetic and orthotic devices.

O&P professionals may work in both orthotics and prosthetics, or they may choose to specialize in one area. Orthotists are specifically trained to work with medical supportive devices, such as braces and inserts. Prosthetists are specifically trained to work with prostheses, such as artificial limbs and other body parts. Some O&P professionals may construct devices for their patients. Others supervise the construction of the orthotic or prosthetic devices by medical appliance technicians.

Orthotists and prosthetists need at least a master's degree and certification before entering the field. Both orthotists and prosthetists must complete a 1-year residency before they can be certified. To learn more, visit http://www.oandp.org.

Phlebotomy: Phlebotomists draw blood for tests, transfusions, research, or blood donations. They also provide assistance if patients have adverse reactions after their blood is drawn. Duties include:

- Drawing blood from patients and blood donors.
- Verifying a patient or donor's identity to ensure proper labeling.
- Entering patient information into an onsite database.
- Assembling and maintaining medical instruments such as needles, test tubes, and blood vials.

Phlebotomists primarily draw blood, which is then used for different kinds of medical laboratory testing. In medical and diagnostic laboratories, patient interaction is often only with the phlebotomist. Because all blood samples look the same, phlebotomists must identify and label the sample they have drawn and enter it into a database. Some phlebotomists draw blood for other purposes, such as at blood drives where people donate blood. To avoid causing infection or other complications, phlebotomists must keep their work area and instruments clean and sanitary.

Phlebotomists typically enter the occupation with a postsecondary non-degree award from a phlebotomy program. Programs for phlebotomy are available from community colleges, vocational schools, or technical schools. These programs usually take less than one year to complete and lead to a certificate or diploma. To learn more about phlebotomy, visit http://www. aspt.org.

Podiatry: Podiatrists provide medical and surgical care for people with foot, ankle, and lower leg problems. They diagnose illnesses, treat injuries, and perform surgery involving the lower extremities. Duties include:

- Assessing the condition of a patient's feet, ankles, or lower legs by reviewing medical history, listening to the patient's concerns, and performing a physical examination.
- Diagnosing foot, ankle, and lower-leg problems through physical exams, x rays, medical laboratory tests, and other methods.
- Providing treatment for foot, ankle, and lower leg ailments, such as prescribing special shoe inserts (orthotics) to improve a patient's mobility.
- Performing foot and ankle surgeries, such as removing bone spurs and correcting foot and ankle deformities.
- Giving advice and instruction on foot and ankle care and on wellness techniques
- Prescribing medications.
- Referring patients to other physicians or specialists if they detect larger health problems, such as diabetes.

Podiatrists treat a variety of foot and ankle ailments, including calluses, ingrown toenails, heel spurs, and arch problems. They also treat foot and leg problems associated with diabetes and other diseases. Some podiatrists spend most of their time performing advanced surgeries, such as foot and ankle reconstruction. Others may choose a specialty such as sports medicine or pediatrics. Podiatrists must earn a Doctor of Podiatric Medicine (DPM) degree and complete a 3-year residency program before they are licensed. For more information and a list of podiatric colleges, visit www.aacpm.org.

Recreational Therapy: Recreational therapists plan, direct, and coordinate recreation-based treatment programs for people with disabilities, injuries, or illnesses. Recreational therapists use a variety of modalities, including arts and crafts, drama, music, dance, sports, games, and community reintegration field trips to help maintain or improve a patient's physical, social, and emotional well-being. Duties include:

- Assessing patients' needs through observations, medical records, tests, and talking with other healthcare professionals, patients' families, and patients.
- Creating treatment plans and programs that meet patients' needs and interests.
- Planning and implementing interventions to prevent harm to a patient.
- Engaging patients in therapeutic activities, such as games and field trips.
- Helping patients learn social skills needed to become or remain independent.
- Teaching patients about ways to cope with anxiety or depression.
- Recording and analyzing a patient's progress.
- Evaluating interventions for effectiveness.

Recreational therapists help people reduce depression, stress, and anxiety, recover basic physical and mental abilities, build confidence, and socialize effectively. They use activities, such as arts and crafts, dance, or sports, to help their patients. Therapists may also provide interventions to patients who need help developing new social and coping skills. For example, a therapist may introduce a therapy dog to patients who need help managing their depression or anxiety. Therapists often work with physicians or surgeons, registered nurses, psychologists, social workers, physical therapists, teachers, or occupational therapists.

Recreational therapists typically need a bachelor's degree. Many employers require therapists to be certified by the National Council for Therapeutic Recreation Certification (NCTRC). For more information, visit http://www.atra-online.com.

Respiratory Therapy: Respiratory therapists care for patients who have trouble breathing—for example, from a chronic respiratory disease, such as asthma or emphysema. Their patients range from premature infants with undeveloped lungs to elderly patients who have diseased lungs. They also provide emergency care to patients suffering from heart attacks, drowning, or shock. Duties include:

- Interviewing and examining patients with breathing or cardiopulmonary disorders
- Consulting with physicians to develop patient treatment plans.
- Performing diagnostic tests such as measuring lung capacity.
- Treating patients by using a variety of methods, including chest physiotherapy and aerosol medications.
- Monitoring and recording the progress of treatment.
- Supervising respiratory therapy technicians during tests and evaluate the findings of the tests.
- Teaching patients how to use treatments.

Respiratory therapists who work in home care teach patients and their families to use ventilators and other life-support systems in their homes. During these visits, they may inspect and clean equipment, check the home for environmental hazards, and ensure that patients know how to use their medications. Therapists also make emergency home visits when necessary. In some hospitals, respiratory therapists are involved in related areas, such as diagnosing breathing problems for people with sleep apnea and counseling people on how to stop smoking. To become a respiratory therapist, you typically need an associate degree, but some have bachelor's degrees, and must be licensed in all states except Alaska. To learn more about respiratory therapy, visit http://aarc.org.

Speech Language Pathology: Speech-language pathologists (sometimes called speech therapists) assess, diagnose, treat, and help to prevent communication and swallowing disorders in patients. Speech, language, and swallowing disorders result from a variety of causes, such as a stroke, brain injury, hearing loss, developmental delay, a cleft palate, cerebral palsy, or emotional problems. Duties include:

- Communicating with patients to evaluate their levels of speech or language difficulty.
- Determining the extent of communication problems by having a patient complete basic reading and vocalizing tasks or by giving standardized tests.
- Identifying treatment options.
- Creating and carrying out an individualized treatment plan.
- Teaching alternative communication methods, such as sign language.
- Working with patients to develop and strengthen the muscles used to swallow.

- Counseling patients and families on how to cope with communication disorders.

Speech-language pathologists work with patients who may be unable to speak at all, or they may speak with difficulty or have rhythm and fluency problems, such as stuttering. They may work with those who are unable to understand language or with people who have voice disorders, such as inappropriate pitch or a harsh voice. Some speech-language pathologists specialize in working with specific age groups, such as children or the elderly. Others focus on treatment programs for specific communication or swallowing problems, such as those resulting from strokes or cleft palate. In medical facilities, speech-language pathologists work with physicians and surgeons, social workers, psychologists, and other healthcare workers. In schools, they work with teachers, other school personnel, and parents to develop and carry out individual or group programs, provide counseling, and support classroom activities.

Speech-language pathologists typically need at least a master's degree. They must be licensed in most states, and the requirements vary by state. To learn more about speech-language pathology, visit http://www.asha.org.

Surgical Technology: Surgical technologists, also called operating room technicians, assist in surgical operations. They prepare operating rooms, arrange equipment, and help doctors during surgeries. Duties include:

- Preparing operating rooms for surgery.
- Sterilizing equipment and making sure that there are adequate supplies for surgery.
- Preparing patients for surgery by washing and disinfecting incision sites.
- Helping surgeons during surgery by passing them instruments and other supplies.
- Counting supplies such as sponges and instruments to maintain sterile environments.

Surgical technologists work as members of a healthcare team alongside physicians and surgeons, registered nurses, and other healthcare workers. Before an operation, surgical technologists prepare the operating room by setting up surgical instruments and equipment. They also prepare patients for surgery by washing and disinfecting incision sites, positioning patients on the operating table, covering patients with sterile drapes, and taking patients to and from the operating room. Surgical technologists prepare sterile solutions and medications used in surgery and check that all surgical equipment is working properly. They help the surgical team put on sterile gowns and gloves. Once the operation is complete, surgical technologists may apply bandages and other dressings to the incision site. They may also help transfer patients to recovery rooms and restock operating rooms after a procedure.

Surgical technologists typically need a postsecondary certificate or an associate degree. A small number of states regulate surgical technologists. To learn more about a career as a surgical technologist, visit http://www.ast.org.

Veterinary Medicine: Veterinarians care for the health of animals and work to improve public health. They diagnose, treat, and research medical conditions and diseases of pets, livestock, and other animals. Duties include:

- Examining animals to diagnose their health problems.
- Diagnosing and treating animals for medical conditions.
- Treating and dressing wounds.
- Performing surgery on animals.
- Testing for and vaccinating against diseases.
- Operating medical equipment such as x-ray machines.
- Advising animal owners about general care, medical conditions, and treatments.
- Prescribing medication.
- Euthanizing animals.

Veterinarians in private clinical practices treat the injuries and illnesses of pets and other animals with a variety of medical equipment, including surgical tools and x-ray and ultrasound machines. They diagnose a variety of diseases and provide treatment for animals that is similar to the services a physician provides to treat humans. The following are examples of types of veterinarians:

Companion animal veterinarians: treat pets and generally work in private clinics and hospitals. According to the American Veterinary Medical Association, more than 75 percent of veterinarians who work in private clinical practice treat pets. They most often care for cats and dogs, but also treat other pets, such as birds, ferrets, and rabbits. These veterinarians diagnose and provide treatment for animal health problems, consult with owners of animals about preventative health care, and carry out medical and surgical procedures, such as vaccinations, dental work, and setting fractures.

Equine veterinarians: work with horses. In 2015, about 8 percent of private practice veterinarians diagnosed and treated horses.

Food animal veterinarians: work with farm animals such as pigs, cattle, and sheep. In 2015, about 10 percent of private practice veterinarians treated food animals. They spend much of their time at farms and ranches treating illnesses and injuries and testing for and vaccinating against disease. They may advise owners or managers about feeding, housing, and general health practices.

Food safety and inspection veterinarians: inspect and test livestock and animal products for major animal illnesses and diseases, provide vaccines to treat animals, enhance animal welfare, conduct research to improve animal health, and enforce government food safety regulations. They design and administer animal and public health programs for the prevention and control of diseases transmissible among animals and between animals and people.

Research veterinarians: work in laboratories, conducting clinical research on human and animal health problems. These veterinarians may perform tests on animals to identify the effects of drug therapies, or they may test new surgical techniques. They may also research how to prevent, control, and eliminate food- and animal-borne illnesses and diseases.

Veterinarians must have a Doctor of Veterinary Medicine degree from an accredited veterinary college and a state license. For more information about veterinary medicine, career opportunities, and a list of U.S. veterinary schools, visit the American Veterinary Medicine Association at www.avma.org.

Professional School Prerequisites and Admissions Requirements

To be accepted as a student in a health professional school, other than medical school, you need to take an admissions exam similar to the MCAT. The following are four alternative options, and educational requirements, for students who decide to choose a career other than medicine:

Dental School

Dentists must be licensed in all states, and the requirements vary by state. To qualify for a license in most states, applicants must graduate from an accredited dental school and pass written and practical exams. In addition, a dentist who wants to practice in one of the nine specialties must have a license in that specialty. This usually requires 2 to 4 years of additional education after dental school and, in some cases, completion of a state exam. A postgraduate residency term also may be required, usually lasting up to 2 years.

Prerequisites: As with medical school, you do not have to major in science, but you must take the DAT and complete the pre-dental science requirements. These include:

- 8 hours Biology with lab
- 8 hours Physics with lab
- 8 hours General Chemistry with lab
- 8 hours Organic Chemistry with lab
- 8 hours English

Dental Admissions Test (DAT): Applicants typically take the DAT a year prior to admission. This is a computerized test that measures academic knowledge, science comprehension, and perceptual ability. It's recommended that you complete your biology and your general and organic chemistry courses before taking the DAT.

Applying: Most U.S. dental schools participate in the Associated American Dental Schools Application Service (AADSAS), which is similar to the AMCAS. Admission is based on GPA, DAT, letters of recommendation, dental office shadowing experiences, and personal interviews. To get a list of U.S. dental schools and to register for the AADSAS, go to the American Dental Education Association at http://www.adea.org/AADSAS.

Optometry School

Optometrists must complete a Doctor of Optometry (O.D.) degree program and obtain a license to practice in a particular state. Doctor of Optometry programs take 4 years to complete, and most students have a bachelor's degree before entering an O.D. program. Some states require individuals to pass an additional clinical exam or an exam on law. All states require optometrists to take continuing education and to renew their license periodically. Optometrists who wish to demonstrate an advanced level of knowledge may choose to become certified by the American Board of Optometry.

Prerequisites: Each optometry school has different prerequisites, so you need to examine their catalogues for specific requirements. In most cases, the prerequisites are similar to those for dental school. At a minimum, you need courses in biology, general chemistry, organic chemistry, and mathematics. Some optometry programs require one semester of organic, while others require two. Check with the school for details.

Optometry Admission Test (OAT): To take the OAT, you must register online at https://www.ada.org/OAT/register.asp. Once your application is processed, you will receive an e-mail notification of eligibility for testing with instructions for appointment scheduling. Tests are administered year-round at test centers in the United States and its territories, including Guam, Puerto Rico, the U.S. Virgin Islands, and Canada.

Applying: Each school has its own application process, admissions requirements, and deadlines, so you'll need to contact each individual school for information. Most schools, however, require the following:

- Their own application forms.
- Optometry Admission Test (OAT) scores.
- Letters of recommendation.
- A personal statement from you about why you chose their school and why you want to become an optometrist.
- A personal interview.
- Demonstrated experience or exposure to the field of optometry.

When you apply to any school, make sure that it's accredited by the Association of Schools and Colleges of Optometry (ASCO). There are only 24 optometry schools in the United States, so if you don't graduate from one of these, you can't be licensed to practice in any state. For more information about optometry, and a list of accredited optometry programs, visit http://www.opted.org.

Pharmacy School

Pharmacists must have a Doctor of Pharmacy (Pharm.D.) degree from an accredited pharmacy program. They also must be licensed, which requires passing licensure and law exams. Pharmacy programs usually take 4 years to finish, although some programs offer a 3-year option. Some schools admit high school graduates into a 6-year program. The North American Pharmacist Licensure Exam (NAPLEX) tests pharmacy skills and knowledge. The Multistate Pharmacy Jurisprudence Exam (MPJE) or a state-specific test on pharmacy law is also required.

Pharmacists may also choose to earn a certification to show their advanced level of knowledge in a certain area. For instance, a pharmacist may become a Certified Diabetes Educator, a qualification offered by the National Certification Board for Diabetes Educators or earn certification in a specialty area, such as nutrition or oncology, from the Board of Pharmacy Specialties. Certifications from both organizations require varying degrees of work experience, as well as passing an exam and paying a fee.

Prerequisites: Admissions requirements vary by program. However all Doctor of Pharmacy programs require that applicants take postsecondary courses such as biology, mathematics, physics, and 2 semesters each of general and organic chemistry. In addition, some schools require biochemistry, microbiology, and anatomy & physiology. You should check each school's catalogue for detailed prerequisites.

Pharmacy College Admission Test (PCAT): Most pharmacy programs require applicants to take the Pharmacy College Admissions Test or PCAT, a computer-based test that is designed specifically for colleges of pharmacy and measures general academic ability and scientific knowledge necessary for a pharmaceutical education. Seating is on a first-come, first-served basis, so register online early at http://www.pcatweb.info/Register-and-Schedule.php.

Applying: Since all schools differ in their application and admission requirements, check with each school that you are interested in for specific details. The American Association of Colleges of Pharmacy at http://www.aacp.org has a list of all pharmacy schools by state. Each school's profile includes its prerequisites and data on accepted applicants such as expected GPA, minimum GPA considered, minimum PCAT scores considered, and other relevant information.

Veterinary School

Veterinarians must complete a Doctor of Veterinary Medicine (D.V.M. or V.M.D.) degree at an accredited college of veterinary medicine. There are currently 32 colleges with accredited programs in the United States. A veterinary medicine program generally takes 4 years to complete and includes classroom, laboratory, and clinical components. The American Veterinary Medical Association offers certification in 40 specialties, such as surgery, microbiology, and internal medicine. Although certification is not required for veterinarians, it can show exceptional skill and expertise in a particular field. To sit for the certification exam, veterinarians must have a certain number of years of experience in the field, complete additional education, and complete a residency program, typically lasting 3 to 4 years. Requirements vary by specialty.

Prerequisites: Although prerequisites vary from school to school, most programs require the VCAT and the following courses:

- 8 hours Biology with lab
- 8 hours Physics with lab
- 8 hours General Chemistry with lab

- 8 hours Organic Chemistry with lab
- 4 hours Biochemistry
- 4 hours Microbiology with lab
- 6 hours Mathematics

Veterinary College Admission Test: The VCAT assesses knowledge and academic ability that is necessary for successful completion of a graduate education in a veterinary college. It is based on approximately 300 total questions in a multiple-choice format, and the questions are independent from any other question unless specifically stated otherwise. The approximate time of the VCAT (including rest and lunch breaks) is about three- and one-half hours. Areas of Testing on the VCAT include: fifty biology questions, fifty chemistry (inorganic and organic) questions, forty reading comprehension questions, forty quantitative questions, and fifty verbal questions.

Applying: Because there are only 32 U.S. veterinary schools, admission to veterinary programs is extremely competitive, and fewer than half of all applicants are usually accepted. When deciding whom to admit, some veterinary medical colleges weigh experience heavily. Formal experience, such as work with veterinarians or scientists in clinics, agribusiness, research, or some area of health science, is particularly advantageous. Less formal experience, such as working with animals on a farm, at a stable, or in an animal shelter, can also be helpful.

CHAPTER 13

STUDY, LEARNING & TEST-TAKING SKILLS

Making the decision to become the best student you can be is the most important first step in getting better grades and improving your chances of getting into medical school. Students are always amazed at how simple it is to study, memorize, learn, and get good grades on virtually any type of exam. Once you learn these effective study techniques, you'll become so confident in your abilities that you will no longer worry about C's and instead concentrate on getting A's. If your goal is to become a physician, you must form excellent study habits and prepare yourself to be a lifelong learner.

No one is born with study skills; you learn them, either by observing others or by being taught them with the help of good teachers. As a college professor and advisor, I've seen students with great potential ruin their chances of getting into select colleges or professional programs simply because they never learned the skills needed to get good grades. I knew these students were smarter than their grades indicated; and given the chance, they would have been successful. As with anything else in life, you're rewarded for hard work and perseverance. Learning to study and take tests effectively will make that work a lot easier.

How to Pay Attention

For many students, the greatest challenge of the school day is getting to class and keeping their minds from thinking about anything but the topic being discussed. The distractions students face today can be overwhelming. Unless there's a problem such as ADD or ADHD, paying attention can become a habit that is easily developed and becomes stronger the more it's done. And like every other habit acquired over a lifetime, this one will become ingrained for life.

Habits are behavior patterns that become regular or spontaneous the more they are repeated. Over time, they become powerful conditioned responses that are incorporated into your subconscious and are triggered whenever you study or receive a mental cue. Like any conditioned reflex, habits are influenced by behaviors and actions, and especially by how often they're performed. Similarly, paying attention is enhanced by mental conditioning and becomes a habit as spontaneous as foot tapping or nail biting. The more you try to concentrate and pay attention, the easier it gets and the more spontaneous it will become. Eventually, listening and paying attention becomes an ingrained, spontaneous habit that is part of your normal behavior pattern.

Virtually any student can develop the habit of paying attention if he or she follows a few simple strategies. Here are four proven ways to do that:

1. **Remind yourself to focus.** Watch a sporting event and you'll see players giving themselves a pep talk. Using words or sentences to help you focus is a good way to direct your actions and help you pay attention. Be positive. For example, remind yourself to keep your eyes focused on the board while the instructor is explaining a topic. Make this a habit and you'll be able to concentrate much better.
2. **Stop negative self-talk.** Many students talk to themselves when they're studying or listening to lectures, but the self-talk is negative. This leads to a negative attitude about school and about one's abilities. For example, don't ever say things like "it's hopeless," or "this is impossible." Instead, be positive and say, "I can do this," or "this is easy." Positive reinforcement feeds on itself and will improve your attitude and your confidence.
3. **Ask questions.** Asking questions while listening to a lecture or while studying really helps focus your attention. For example, when reading about World War II, you might ask yourself, "Which countries did Germany occupy? Which were our friends and allies? Who did Germany fight with?" As you're reading, you can also ask yourself what the paragraph was about, what the main point was, etc.

   Asking questions during a lecture does not need to be verbal. As the instructor is lecturing, question the things he or she is saying or writing. This is especially effective if you read the material beforehand and anticipate what the lecture will be about. Asking questions serves two purposes: it helps bring your wandering mind back to the task at hand, and it helps you to remember what's being said because you become involved in the process.
4. **Set specific study goals.** Setting goals specific to the topic you're studying helps your attention span. One goal might be to study a short lesson until you can explain the main point; another might be to solve a math problem, or to know specific names, dates, and places. Many smaller goals are more effective in helping you stay focused than one larger goal.

A wandering mind is overcome easily by reconditioning your brain to replace wandering with concentration. The key to reconditioning is to use techniques such as the ones described to force you into replacing a bad habit with a good one. Once you've done that, learning and studying will become surprisingly easy and very rewarding.

Developing Learning and Study Skills

We all learn by a combination of seeing, hearing, and doing. But by adjusting some of your study habits to fit your dominant learning style, you'll be much more successful in your classes. For instance, if you're a visual learner, draw lots of diagrams and charts in your notes, make lists, and use colored highlighters. If you're an auditory learner, study by reading out loud, forming a study group with other students, participating in discussions, asking lots of questions, etc. And if you're a kinesthetic learner (hands on and physical), take more lab courses, study with others so that you can lecture to them, take a few more breaks so that you don't get burned out, etc.

The days when students were expected to study and learn only one way are long gone. Teachers realize that everyone is different, and that each student learns in his/her own unique way. To be the most successful student you can be, recognize what your learning style is and then change your study habits to reflect that style. The first step in improving learning skills is managing and organizing the information given to you. This could be difficult if the instructor is not good at organizing his or her material to begin with. But if you have the organizational tools needed to overcome a poor lecture, it should not really matter. The following are four ways to enhance learning in any class you take.

1. **Familiarize yourself with the lecture material beforehand.** By knowing something about the topic, you'll recognize key ideas and words when you hear them. This will help you concentrate on what's being said rather than worrying about not understanding the material. If you cannot read over the material, at least skim through it to get the main points.
2. **As soon as possible after class, rewrite your notes in a clear and organized manner.** In all my years as a teacher, I've seen few unedited notes that I would study from. Many students' notes are a jumble of disorganized sentences and missing words. This is where rewriting is important. You can fill in missing information, clear up gaps, eliminate clutter, and add material. The physical act of reading and rewriting your notes also reinforces what you have heard and is an excellent way to learn the material while it's still fresh in your mind. Always keep the clean, edited version at home as a safeguard against loss and take your regular notebook to class.
3. **Use folders and files to organize study materials.** Besides using a class notebook, develop a system for filing papers, articles, and handouts that will be available whenever you need them. A file system prevents a lot of wasted effort looking for study materials before exams, and it will get you in the habit of becoming more organized and efficient.
4. **Make flash cards for things like formulas, equations, dates, definitions, etc.** If you must memorize material, write it down on index cards. Every week or so, go through your flash cards until you have the material memorized. Change the order of cards each time you review, and study them backwards and forwards in case the question is asked in a different way. Teachers will often word exams differently to make sure you know the material.

A key step in improving study and learning skills is by taking the material you've organized and inputting it into your brain in the simplest way possible. Once mastered, this skill will enable you to retrieve any information you are given in class. The fact is that

95 percent of the most important information in a textbook can be located quickly because authors and publishers who know what they're doing offer roadmaps within each chapter. Learning to pick through written material, and finding the important details you need, will make studying that much easier.

Studying is more than just sitting down at a desk, opening your notebook, and reading your notes. It takes planning. Students waste a lot of time and effort because they don't realize that the amount of time spent studying is not as important as the way they spend their time studying. It's like being in the gym and watching two people work out. One spends 30 minutes training effectively, building muscle and losing fat, while the other spends two hours wasting time and never getting results. Studying is the same. Even 30 minutes of effective study is better than 4 hours of poor study.

One of the biggest complaints I hear from students is that there's not enough time in the day to do all their work. That's nonsense. Anyone can develop effective study and learning skills and have plenty of time in their day for schoolwork. If that were not true, how can so many students work a full-time job and still get good grades? Here are seven things you can do that will guarantee results.

1. **Find your best study time.** Because we all have unique biological clocks, we function differently during various times of the day. Some of us are morning people, some night owls. Our individual biological clocks dictate whether we are better off studying when we first get up in the morning or whether we are better off waiting until later in the evening. Although you can train yourself to study at any time, you should find when your peak energy levels are so that you can make the most of that energy for maximum learning.
2. **Manage your time efficiently.** Part of effective learning is time management. To study well, establish a schedule and a study routine. Like habits, routines become ingrained and, once established, are easy to follow. Write down a daily or weekly schedule, which includes times for study, relaxation, or seeing friends. Schedules should be flexible, allowing shifting for work, chores, or other plans, as long as the shifting does not become constant and disruptive.
3. **Never study more than an hour at a time without a break.** The average person begins to lose concentration after about an hour. A serious mistake that students make is cramming or studying too long at any one time. Instead of absorbing information, you'll be wasting a lot of time and effort because your brain is not capable of maintaining a high level of concentration without a break ever so often. The rule should be to take a ten-minute break every hour or so. It's also a good idea to switch subjects between learning sessions because studies have found that studying the same subject for prolonged periods of time can decrease your concentration and your ability to learn.
4. **Make your study space conducive to study.** To ensure successful learning, avoid distractions. If you know that certain times will be especially noisy or active, eliminate them from your study schedule. Instead, schedule your study during

periods of the day or evening you know will be most peaceful. Also, make sure you have plenty of bright light because memory, concentration, and positive attitude are enhanced when you're exposed to light, especially natural daylight.

5. **Avoid foods that prevent learning.** If possible, don't eat simple carbohydrates, especially junk food, before or during your study sessions. While carbohydrates are a prime source of energy, simple sugars will cause a sudden insulin spike and then make you crash. The last thing you want to do is settle in for a nap in the middle of studying. Also, give up habits that prevent your brain from reaching its full potential, and that is smoking and excessive drinking.
6. **Form a study group.** Being actively involved with other students and discussing study material will help you concentrate and absorb the material better. An added advantage is that someone in the study group will have information you may have missed or written down incorrectly. During your study sessions, ask one another questions, take mock exams, and teach one another. According to studies, we learn only 10% of what we read but 70% of what we discuss and 90% of what we teach to others.

The way in which you study will make a big difference in how much you learn. Paying attention, managing and organizing class notes, and conditioning your brain to concentrate are all important. But for many students, the technique of questioning is one of the best ways to enhance learning. Study routines should always include questioning, either by yourself as a means of self-evaluation or by fellow students who are studying with you. Just as important, however, is to learn to ask yourself better questions; questions that lead to more and even deeper questions, as well as answers.

Even before Socrates, who repeatedly asked his students questions as a way of teaching, questioning was a common learning strategy. Some questions require only factual recall without much thought or analysis; others are thought-provoking and force you to think on a deeper level. These are the types of questions that make you learn.

There's a big difference between your asking "When did Lincoln deliver his Gettysburg Address?" and "Why was Lincoln's Gettysburg Address an important speech?" Each question has its place, but the second one makes you analyze the speech in terms of the issues surrounding the Civil War. The second question makes you think and really enhances learning. Here are some effective strategies for using questioning as a study tool:

1. **When reading, ask yourself questions to find the main point.** For example, if you're reading about immigration patterns from different countries, ask questions about important issues such as "Why are these people immigrating? From which countries are they coming? How are their lives being changed? How is their immigration affecting the country they are immigrating to?" It's also a good strategy to ask the general question, "What's the point here?" All this questioning will help you focus on what you're reading and force you to study actively rather than passively.
2. **Discuss material with other students.** Being actively involved by forming study

groups and discussing topics forces you to concentrate on the material. Therefore study sessions and study groups are so effective. Someone in the study group will always come up with a thought-provoking question or look at something in a way that no one else had thought of. Discussing makes you think; and taking advantage of the group's participation and total knowledge is a great way to absorb information.

3. **Immediately after a lecture, write down important questions about the topic and then answer them.** This technique forces you to think about what you did and did not understand about the lecture. Ask yourself questions like "What's the most important thing I learned today?" "What didn't I understand about the lecture?" "What can I do to help me understand the material better?" "How can I explain in my own words what I learned today?"

Note-Taking

Unless you have a photographic memory, it's impossible to remember everything you hear in a lecture. Besides, speakers have quite different lecture styles. Some are prepared, well-organized, and crystal clear; others drone on, get off topic, or are so boring that you must force your eyelids to stay open. Good notetaking can often compensate for a poor lecture. It helps you focus on the material and select the information that is important rather than trying to write down every word being said.

The purpose of taking notes is to help you outline critical ideas and main points, especially those that the lecturer thinks are important. Taking notes forces you to listen more carefully. Because they are a summary of what you just spent an hour listening to, they need to be legible, efficient, and concise. A good note-taker prepares for the lecture beforehand, uses effective note-taking techniques during the lecture, and then reviews and rewrites notes after the lecture. Good notetaking helps you use in-class time wisely and get the most out of every lecture.

The most important note-taking strategy happens before you even walk into a lecture. Nothing is more frustrating than not understanding what a teacher is talking about or frantically trying to write down every word the teacher says. At the end of the lecture, you walk out with pages of notes but have little understanding of what they mean because you were too busy writing instead of listening. Here are some tips on what to do before a lecture to make notetaking as efficient as possible:

1. **Read and review the material beforehand.** Getting a general feel for what a lecture will be about is half the battle. By having at least some knowledge of the material, you will be able to concentrate better during the lecture, anticipate important concepts and ideas, and will not be scrambling to write down every word the instructor is saying.
2. **Familiarize yourself with key words and concepts.** As you read, jot down unfamiliar terms and then look them up before class. When you hear them during the lecture, you'll recognize them and will not be so distracted.
3. **Bring a list of questions.** Once you've read the chapter, write down some questions

you might want to ask the instructor. Listen for the answers and explanations during the lecture; and if your questions are not answered, ask them at the end.

Regardless of the note-taking system you use, they all have one thing in common: to provide you with an easy-to-read outline of information you'll need to study, review, and learn. But you also need to be flexible. Change your note-taking system to fit various lecture types, or if it's not working for you. The bottom line is that your notetaking must help you learn and result in better grades.

What you do immediately after class, or at least within 24 hours of the lecture, is just as important as what you do before or during a lecture. In fact, experts on learning and study skills consider post lecture review and editing the most important part of learning. The following suggestions will enhance the notes you take and significantly increase your ability to learn the material.

- **Edit anything that is not legible.** Within a day of the lecture, sit down and go over your notes. Correct inconsistencies, fix errors, add key word, include details, and clean up illegible writing while the material is still fresh in your mind. The longer you wait, the harder it is to remember what you have written. If necessary, talk to your instructor, your classmates, or consult your textbook and additional sources to clear things up.
- **Review the material.** Retention falls off sharply the longer you wait to review. So within 24 hours, go over your lecture notes so that you're not relearning material that you should be reviewing. This is also where a stack of index cards comes in handy. By periodically using flash cards to review, you will always keep the material fresh in your mind.
- **Rewrite your notes.** Some experts say that rewriting notes is not necessary, but I don't think it's ever a waste of time to rewrite your notes. I did it for every one of my classes. In fact, the very act of rewriting is really your first review. If you're going to spend several hours studying from your notes anyway, why not add an extra dimension to your learning? If nothing else, rewriting is active learning. It gets you involved more than simply reading or editing. Finally, a clean set of notes without a lot of marks, smudges, lines and cross-outs will make study easier because you will not have to fight through a maze of corrections.

Recall and Memorization

Most of us have spent a lot of extra hours studying for an exam simply because we had problems memorizing the material. Whether you like it or not, certain subjects like Anatomy, History, and Geography require you to recall details, names, numbers, facts, dates, or other information. The good news is that memorizing these things is a learned skill. The more you try to remember things, the more you exercise your brain and the easier it will be to remember the next time. Developing a system for memorizing will jump start your study sessions and make your school life a lot easier.

One of the most important elements in memory is the ability to observe. Without observation, we have nothing to input into our brain. Imagine a detective at the scene of a crime who walks into a room and only looks at the body of the victim without noticing anything else around him. He would go back to the precinct and not have very much to report other than that the victim was lying in the middle of the room. The same thing often happens when you read or try to memorize something. You might get through an entire page, only to realize that you have no idea what you had just read. Maybe you were thinking about something else, or listening to a song on the radio, or watching a TV show. Whatever it was, it was enough of a distraction that your mind was not focused, and you missed the point of what you were reading.

To improve your observational skills and, therefore, your memory, all you need to do is make a conscious effort to observe. It sounds simple, but many students really need to do this to prevent thinking about other things and having their minds wander. Tell yourself beforehand that you're going to observe. Unless you make a real effort to observe everything, no memories will form that link to what you're trying to learn.

The term mnemonic comes from a Greek word meaning to remember. It is any device that helps us recall information, and it could be a word, a short phrase, a list, a song, or even a visual or auditory cue. Mnemonics rely on links between what we already know and what we need to remember. This is based on the principle that our mind can more easily remember personal, physical, sexual, exaggerated, vivid, or humorous information than more arbitrary or abstract things.

One of the problems we face when we study is that our brains have evolved a way of interpreting and storing stimuli like smell, taste, touch, vision, and hearing, but when it comes to remembering words on paper, it doesn't do as well. The other problem is that some of us are either right-brained or left-brained, which makes it difficult to remember certain subjects because we are not naturally inclined to find those subjects easy to learn. Along comes mnemonics, which uses the brain's ability to interpret difficult-to-remember information to help us remember just about anything. Here are ways to make mnemonics much more effective:

- **Make your images move.** Actions trigger memory more so than any static image can. When you try to memorize something, make it move, give it life, and add some zest to your images.
- **Use colors to stimulate the senses.** Color is a great stimulant, so try to imagine things in color rather than in black and white.
- **Make your images funny or ridiculous.** The funnier, bizarre, sexy, and/or more ridiculous you make your image, the more likely you will remember it. Add some action to the funny image and it will be even more memorable.
- **Exaggerate size and shape.** Make your images bigger than life or exaggerate one or more of the main features. This goes hand in hand with the previous suggestion of making your images funny, bizarre, or ridiculous.

- **Use all your senses.** The best mnemonics are ones that contain movements, smells, sounds, tastes, and feelings. Your senses are powerful tools that can condition your brain to remember things and then trigger recall.

For a mnemonic device to work well for a specific topic, and be as powerful as it can be, use ideas and images from your own personal experiences and make good use of your imagination. Think back to your childhood and remember how much fun it was to imagine silly things. Imagination creates images that are memorable, and if you use images that are familiar to you they will be much stronger and even more memorable.

Probably the simplest way to remember something is to use a device we're all familiar with ever since we started school, and that is to use a sentence with the first letter of each word acting as a cue for what you need to remember. These devices have been standard memory techniques for many years because they're simple, and they work.

One example would be if you wanted to remember that the steps of cell division, in order, are: **I**nterphase, **P**rophase, **M**etaphase, **A**naphase, and **T**elophase. In this case, just make a sentence like **I** **P**ray **M**ondays **A**nd **T**uesdays. To remember the order of the planets **M**ercury, **V**enus, **E**arth, **M**ars, **J**upiter, **S**aturn, **U**ranus, **N**eptune, **P**luto, you might use a sentence like **M**y **V**ery **E**xcited **M**other **J**ust **S**erved **U**s **N**ine **P**ickles. Or how about in taxonomy, when you need to remember **K**ingdom, **P**hylum, **C**lass, **O**rder, **F**amily, **G**enus, **S**pecies? You might use a sentence like **K**ing **P**hilip **C**uts **O**pen **F**ive **G**reen **S**nakes.

Another effective method is to use a single word as an acronym, with each letter representing the idea you must recall. For example, **BRASS** may be the acronym for the steps you need to go through when shooting a rifle: **B**reath, **R**elax, **A**im, **S**ight, and **S**queeze. If you need to remember the five Great Lakes, which are Huron, Ontario, Michigan, Erie, and Superior, use a word likes **HOMES**. Of course everyone knows that **FACE** represents musical notes on the spaces between lines. Whatever system you choose, make sure it is one that you will remember easily. Sometimes a common word is not as effective as one that sounds strange or is somehow related to what you're trying to memorize. Use your imagination and go with what works best for you.

Of all the senses in your body, the sense of sight is the most responsive you have. In fact, for most students, the information they remember best is information they see, not what they hear. So to add permanence to your memory, you need to produce vivid mental images that will be ingrained in your mind. The two important rules to follow for effective visualization are to make your images as vivid and as exaggerated as possible, and to make them animated.

A great way to remember facts is to come up with an image you will associate with the fact. For example, how would you remember that Frankfort is the capital of Kentucky? The first thing to do is search your knowledge base. You know that Kentucky is known as the bluegrass state and is famous for thoroughbred racehorses. So, if you want to remember that Frankfort is the capital city of Kentucky, picture in your mind a big, fat, giant frankfurter inside a bun grazing on a blue pasture next to thoroughbreds.

The more ridiculous the picture is the better. Try it. Close your eyes and imagine a hot dog the size of a horse grazing on blue grass. Keep that image in your mind a few seconds and then forget it. A week later, ask yourself what the capital of Kentucky is, and that image will pop into your head immediately.

Another memory technique, called the Roman room system, has been around an exceptionally long time. Also called the memory palace or the Loci method, this technique has you create a mental picture of a room, typically your home or any room that you're intimately familiar with and then, as you walk around the room, link items in the room with a list of things you need to remember in no particular order. To recall information, you begin by visualizing the items you know well and linking them with images of whatever it is you need to memorize. The two main rules when using this method are:

1. **Imprint the room and its contents in your mind.** Close your eyes and take some time to really get to know your room. Spend an hour or more if you need to, but make sure that your room is always the same and that the items are in the right places so that the process becomes ingrained.
2. **Make the images you want to remember vivid and active.** The livelier, more exaggerated, and more ridiculous the image you want to remember is, the more likely it will be that you will remember it.

As an example, imagine that your living room has the following items: coffee table, sofa, bookcase, lamp, television, stereo, mirror, and painting. These are you peg images. Let's say that you need to remember that the five classes of vertebrates are fish, amphibians, reptiles, birds, and mammals. As you walk into the living room, you image fish flopping around on your coffee table. You then see two giant frogs sitting and kissing on your sofa. When you look at your bookcase, you see hundreds of snakes slithering out from between the books. Next to the bookcase, you imagine your lamp and see a large eagle flying out from beneath the lampshade. Finally, you look at the television and see several monkeys fighting over the remote control.

The technique works best when the room and the items are familiar to you and if the images are as ridiculous and animated as they can be. You can expand this system by adding doors through which you walk through and go into other rooms that contain more familiar items that you can use as pegs.

An effective way to make new and unfamiliar information more meaningful and more likely to be remembered is through inferences and analogies. This involves thinking about the information, ideas, or opinions and drawing conclusions from that new information. For example, if you're reading about an invention, you might think about how it changed people's lives and habits at the time of the invention. Or when studying the circulatory system, you might think about how diet, activity, or illness can affect it.

Creating inferences force you to think. You become an active rather than a passive learner. And being active in your learning keeps your mind from wandering and enhances your concentration. This, in turn, increases your ability to store information into long-term memory. The very act of making inferences while reading or studying stimulates brain cells and will increase your capacity to learn. Analogies are similarities between things that are otherwise not alike. You create the most effective analogies when you compare new material with material you already know well.

Here's an example: suppose you're trying to learn the differences between arteries in the human body, which are large blood vessels that have great pressure and carry oxygen-rich blood out to the body's organs and tissues, and veins, which are much thinner, have low pressure, and carry oxygen-poor blood back to the heart. One way to think about this is to make a plumbing analogy. Think of the water as blood, the pipes under the sink as veins, the faucet as a heart and arteries, and the sink as the body. The water (blood) comes out of the faucet (heart and arteries) with great force and carries it out to the sink (body). The water (blood) is used in the sink (body), leaves, and drains in the pipes (veins) with much less force before it goes to the water treatment plant and back to the faucet (heart).

Regular review of your study material is essential for proper recall. Even if you become an expert in memory techniques, you still must reinforce the information stored in your memory through periodic review. The following are some proven strategies for using review as a memory tool.

- **Go over lecture material every day or so.** Most of your forgetting occurs shortly after learning has taken place. By not allowing too much time to pass between the time you get the information and the time you review it, you will reinforce what's in your head. Under no circumstances should you go more than a week before reviewing.
- **When reviewing, have a pen or pencil in your hand.** Actively review by jotting down key ideas, principles, concepts, and questions you think might be on the next exam. If necessary, draw diagrams, charts, and illustrations since pictures make the information more vivid and understandable.
- **Have a cumulative review every week.** Each week go back to your class notes and review previous material, which will not only reinforce what you've already learned, it will help you understand new material. Use the flash cards you've been accumulating for additional reinforcement.
- **Read your notes out loud.** When reviewing, use as many of your senses as possible. Information that you input into your brain through both your eyes and your ears is going to be stored more easily than information you only read. That's because your brain is getting the information several ways. Add to that some rewriting and you are really using your senses in the most effective way possible.
- **Categorize review material.** When reviewing large amounts of information, it helps to group it into categories. For example, when reviewing for a Zoology exam, study animals after dividing them into groups such as reptiles, mammals, fish, birds, amphibians, etc. If you're learning about musical instruments, it helps to organize them into strings, brass, woodwinds, and percussion. It's much easier to remember several smaller groups of related items than to remember one large group.
- **Review in short rather than long sessions.** According to new research, memory is

significantly increased when information is spread out over several short days rather than one long day. A famous study found that it took individuals 68 repetitions to remember information they were given, but when spread out over a 3-day period, the individuals needed only 38 repetitions to remember the same information. That's a fifty percent reduction in work.

- **Before exams, lecture to yourself from your notes.** While reviewing, become the teacher and lecture to your imaginary class as you review. Try to imagine that you're explaining the material to students as if they were hearing the information for the first time. Remember, we learn 90% of what we teach to others.

Since most of us are not blessed with super memories, we must rely on techniques and tricks that help our brain remember things. Just like a computer stores data, our brain stores whatever we see and hear; but like a computer, it can hide it from us much like our losing access to one of our computer files. We know it's there; we just can't retrieve it.

Mental hooks, images, and cues are all highly effective in getting at information that we know is inside our brain but needs to be jarred loose. The problem is not that we don't store the information; it's that we cannot access it. The more you use mnemonic techniques and follow the other suggestions for improving memory, the easier it becomes to remember. And once you begin to master the art of recall, your entire attitude about studying and learning will change because you'll discover that memory is not necessarily something you're born with but a skill that you learn.

Improving Reading Skills

College, and especially medical school, requires enormous amounts of reading. Students who improve their reading will dramatically improve their ability to learn and, as a result, automatically improve their grades. Good readers are typically good learners because they can dig down for important information and then process it in their brains. They are also efficient at what they read, gleaning facts and skimming over material that is not as critical. Knowing what to skip over is often just as important because it helps you focus and manage your time.

Unless you have good reading skills, studying math and science, and analyzing problems is next to impossible. But once you become a skillful reader, you will transition from someone who learned to read to someone who reads to learn. So to read more effectively and with more comprehension and understanding, you need to do four things: (1) follow chapter roadmaps, (2) read actively rather than passively, (3) increase reading speed, and (4) enhance your vocabulary to increase comprehension.

Textbook publishers use a format that makes 90 percent of the most important information easy to locate. However, if the material in a chapter is new, you cannot expect to identify and remember the key points or concepts right away. That's like asking you to locate someone's address in a different city without a street map. You have no means of relating the new address to streets you're not familiar with. A map provides you with cues that help you know you're going in the right direction. In the same way, a good textbook provides a map so that you can find your way through sometimes difficult material.

The map is made up of three main sections: An **Introduction**, the **Headings**, and a **Summary**. Sometimes an overview is included at the beginning that explains the purpose of the chapter. The introduction tells you what the chapter will cover, while the summary serves as an outline of the most important material. Here is how to approach each section:

Introduction: Read this section of the chapter carefully. When written well, the introduction gives you a good idea of what's ahead. Pause for a moment after reading it and reflect on what the author's purpose is.

Headings: These are typically bold-faced, capitalized, or both. The headings tell you exactly what the section of the chapter includes and prepares you for the material you are about to read. If there are subheadings, try to link them to the main heading to get a sense of how the material is being presented. Pause between headings and think about the content and what you have finished reading.

Summary: Read the summary as carefully as you did the introduction. Here, the author is repeating or emphasizing his or her ideas, main points or arguments. Pause for a few moments after reading the summary, think about what you've read, and try to incorporate the ideas in the summary with the chapter headings.

Many texts include pictures, charts, graphs, illustrations, and vocabulary terms in bold print. These often do more to help you understand the text than the written material, so don't overlook them. Special type is sometimes placed within the text to draw your attention to important information. Don't ignore this, especially if the type is boldface. If special type attracts your attention, it's because the material is worth going over carefully.

After you preview the chapter and make sure you get a clear picture of what it is you're about to read, you are now in a better position to read actively. One of the most important things you want to do is find relationships between the material you read and your own knowledge base. This is what comprehension is all about.

Use information from the chapter preview to ask yourself questions that you expect to answer. Some students find it useful to pause before each new section of a chapter and use some of the main learning and memory aids, such as analogies, inferences, categorizing information, asking questions, finding main ideas, etc. to help them focus on and remember the material. By creating analogies, making inferences, and asking questions, you know that you're doing more than just skimming the page; you're getting something out of your reading. If you find yourself wondering what you just finished reading, it means that your mind was somewhere other than on what you were reading. Refocus and get back to active reading.

One of the great things about using attention-focusing techniques is that you will be elaborating on what you're reading and then generating connections between what you already know or have experienced and what you read. This makes the material much more understandable and easier to remember because you're not waiting until you finish the entire section to elaborate.

Stopping to elaborate part way through the text is an effective method to increase comprehension and memory, but it also depends on the complexity of the subject. You may need to stop more often when reading a math or science text than you would when reading a history or sociology text. This active reading process is what keeps your mind on the task at hand. Marking a textbook with a pencil or highlighter is an excellent way to help you read actively. Here are some ideas for making notes in your book while you read:

- **Underline main ideas.** Without getting too carried away, use a highlight pen to color important words and phrases. Highlighting is better than underling because it's not as visually distracting.
- **Place asterisks in the margins next to important points.** If the asterisks are drawn in red or blue, they will stand out more and draw your attention to the main points of the text.
- **Place numbers within the text next to lists of main ideas or important points.** When you do this, don't be so sloppy that your numbers cover up important words. Also, use a colored pen or pencil. Colors within the text will be more noticeable, and you will not have to read through the entire text to find a list of main points.
- **Circle new words to be learned.** When you come across new terms, circle them and make sure to look them up as soon as you can. In most cases, understanding the vocabulary terms is related to understanding the reading material.
- **Place notes in margins.** When reading, always have a pen or pencil in hand. The very act of jotting down notes and thoughts in the margins will get you actively involved in the reading process. Later, as you review, the thoughts you may have forgotten will be right there in the text along with the material.

When using these techniques, be careful not to cover up the words. Don't overdo it with the underlining or highlighting. Use too many lines and highlights and the ideas become lost among all the markings. The value of this system pays off when it's time to review because you will not have to reread page after page of text again. All the important information will be right there and easily located. So, make active reading a habit and it will become a natural part of study and learning.

When you first learned to read, your reading comprehension was limited to single words. You associated a word with a sound or an object. As you progressed, you formed words into groups or phrases and then sentences. Once you were able to put those related sentences together to form a single idea within a paragraph, you were well on your way toward reading with comprehension.

Good readers go a step further. They take entire paragraphs and sections and link them together to get an overall understanding of what it is they're reading. To accomplish that, you need to do three things: develop a good workable vocabulary, without which you can't really comprehend complex ideas and topics, recognize how authors are presenting the material, which involves previewing and mapping the chapter, and relate what you're reading to what you already know or have already experienced in other classes or in your own life. Developing a good vocabulary should be an ongoing process that you work on continually.

The second factor in comprehension – recognizing how the author is presenting the material – is important but is often overlooked. Whenever authors write a book, they break it down into introduction, body, and conclusion. Once they get you through the introduction, which should tell you what the chapter is about, authors use the body of the text to describe, explain, or discuss the material before summarizing it. The conclusion or summary is the author's final attempt at making the material clear. When reading the body of a text, here is what to look for:

Examples: Authors like to use various examples, not only to explain the material they're writing about, but also to hold the reader's attention. Look for examples immediately following explanations or discussions. They will reinforce what you read and are often an important part of the book.

Definitions and illustrations: Within the body of the text, authors provide definitions and illustrations to elucidate ideas and main points. Never ignore these. Definitions explain what the author is talking about; and illustrations can be a better way to explain the material than the text itself. I often select textbooks based mainly on the quality of illustrations and how well they relate to the text. So, as you read, pay particular attention to how the author is using an illustration to describe information.

Causes and effects: Whenever you read, try to figure out why something has caused something else to happen. For example, when an author is writing about the collapse of the former Soviet Union, you might ask yourself questions about the events that led up to the collapse or the factors that caused the circumstances leading up to the collapse. Doing this every time you read will make you a critical thinker as well.

Comparisons and contrasts: This technique is similar to making analogies. Authors using this technique are trying to compare what they're writing about to what they think you should already know. For example, when discussing the British system of government, an author may compare it to or contrast it with the American system of government. Pay special attention to this kind of writing.

The third factor in comprehension – relating what you're reading to what you know or have experienced – is a key element of active reading. Ask yourself how the information compares to your experiences or the experiences of others. Also ask yourself what the author is trying to say, what the objectives are, why the author has written the material in this manner, and why the author feels the way he or she does about the material.

By interpreting and analyzing information, you're getting inside the author's head, which is precisely the point of active reading. Whenever you do this, your understanding improves and with it your ability to remember more of what you read.

Some years ago, one of my colleagues pointed out something to me that I found to be almost always true. He told me that a student often misses the main point or the meaning of a sentence because of one unfamiliar word. That one little word makes a student stop dead in his or her tracks and disrupts thought and concentration. It follows then that the better your vocabulary is the better your reading and comprehension will be. On the other hand, the more words you get stuck on as you read, the more frustrated you're going to be and the less you're going to want to continue reading. Vocabulary adds tremendous power to your learning. An added benefit is that you'll do much better on standardized tests, which assume a good knowledge of vocabulary.

There are many ways to improve your vocabulary. Go to any bookstore and you'll find a dozen good books on the subject, each one offering great techniques for learning new words. However, one of the best ways is to invest in a good dictionary and use it often! When you read something, circle, underline, or mark words you don't know. Go back and look up those words.

Another great way to improve your vocabulary is by reading a variety of books and magazines. Don't only read about what you're interested in, and don't avoid certain topics because they're unfamiliar to you. Challenge yourself by reading a wide variety of topics, especially ones you are not familiar with, and your general vocabulary will expand quickly.

Good readers read with both speed and comprehension. They look for ideas, concepts, and main points within sentences and paragraphs, and they condition their eyes to pick up entire blocks of words rather than focusing on single words. They also eliminate habits like rereading and pausing, and they know when to slow down and speed up depending on the different material they're reading. Here are some final suggestions I found personally useful.

- **Spend some of your leisure time reading.** Research shows that the amount of leisure time spent reading is directly related to reading comprehension, the size of your vocabulary, and gains in reading ability. This is especially true if you read a wide variety of subject matter, including fiction and non-fiction. So, instead of watching TV or playing that video game, spend time reading. You'll find that it gets to be an enjoyable habit.
- **Look for signposts as you read.** There are certain words or groups of words that signal you to go ahead or to change direction. Both tell you to look out for upcoming ideas. Some go-ahead signals include: accordingly, also, as a result, furthermore, in conclusion, in fact, in summary, likewise, moreover, and subsequently. Changing direction signals include: although, despite, however, in spite of, on the contrary, notwithstanding, rather, regardless, and yet.

Based on years of teaching, I must agree with many experts who say that without good reading skills students are doomed to mediocrity. If you cannot read effectively, you can't develop the foundation necessary to get good grades. More importantly, you'll not have the ability to learn what you need to know to become successful. It's true that the most successful students have the best reading habits; and if you want to transform yourself into a top student, read well and read often.

Improving Test-Taking Skills

As a teacher for over 30 years, I've had students who should have been getting A's and B's but failed simply because they didn't know how to prepare for and take exams. I've also had average students do much better than I thought they could because they were good test-takers. In many cases, getting good grades on tests is just a matter of knowing how to read and interpret questions.

There's no secret to doing well on exams. Sometimes all it takes is preparation and strategy and using certain techniques for eliminating wrong choices. But the first step is to be prepared. This happens from day one of class by paying attention, taking good notes, keeping up with homework, and using effective study and review techniques. But once you begin to study in earnest, there are certain things you need to do to make your test preparation as good as it can be. Here are some suggestions:

- **Manage your time.** I'm sure you've heard it a thousand times, but I'll say it again. Do not cram for exams! Instead, organize and budget your time, and be studying and reviewing all along. Cramming may work for some students, but for most it's not very effective at all.
- **Use review sessions.** Students who attend regular review sessions, even if they don't need to, typically do much better on exams. Instructors at review sessions will often go over material that will be on exams and give examples of questions that students will expect to see.
- **Practice the material.** Use practice tests, sample problems in the text or in your notes, review materials, and whatever else you can find, to learn the material. The Power Law of Human Performance states that the time it takes an individual to perform a task decreases as the number of times the individual practices that task increases. In other words, your grade will reflect the amount of time you put into your study.
- **Make a review sheet.** Condense exam material to a single sheet with only the main ideas and key concepts. Use this as a guide that you can refer to several times when studying.
- **Get a good night's sleep.** All-nighters are a bad idea if you want to do well, especially if the exam is first thing in the morning. To get a good night's sleep, don't drink alcohol the evening before an exam, and do not eat a heavy meal at least 3 hours before going to bed.
- **Do not go to an exam hungry.** Nothing is worse than a growling stomach and hunger pangs in the middle of a test. So, before your exam, eat a good meal that consists of protein and complex carbs. Avoid simple sugars, which cause an insulin spike, and heavy foods that will make you groggy.
- **Arrive 10 minutes early.** By getting to your exam a little early, you can relax and get yourself mentally prepared. Besides, if you arrive late you might miss any hints or last-minute exam instructions.
- **Arrive prepared.** Always bring extra pens and pencils, erasers, a watch to pace

yourself, and a calculator with fresh batteries.

- **Use the bathroom before an exam.** You don't want to be worrying about bodily functions while trying to concentrate. So, go to the bathroom before you go in to take your exam.
- **Prioritize the exam questions.** Once you get the exam, make a quick survey and answer the questions with the highest point values first. Do the ones you're most certain of, and don't spend time on a question you're stuck on, especially when you're pressed for time. You can always go back. In some cases, other parts of the test will have information that can trigger your memory and help you with a question you could not answer.
- **Learn how to take different types of exams.** There are certain rules and techniques to follow depending on the type of exam you're taking. Here are some suggestions for doing well on different types of exams:

Multiple Choice Questions

Multiple choice tests are the most common tests teachers give, especially in large classes. Students either like them or they don't; and some students are much better at answering multiple choice questions because they know the rules. The following are some tips for taking different types of multiple-choice tests and doing well, even if you're not sure of the answer.

- **Answer the question before looking at the choices.** This strategy is effective if you know the material well. By answering the question and then looking at the multiple-choice answers, you will know that you're correct if you see your answer as one of the choices. Sometimes students get confused when answers seem similar, and this technique can eliminate that.
- **Eliminate wrong answers.** Sometimes you just know when an answer is wrong. By eliminating at least two wrong answers, you'll increase the odds that you will get the correct answer just by guessing. One out of three is much better odds than one out of five.
- **Eliminate extremes.** In math and science courses, usually the correct answer is somewhere in the middle. For example, a biology exam might have the question "What is the pH of blood?" If the answers are: a) 2.0 b) 4.5 c) 6.2 d) 7.4 e) 9.0, eliminate the extremes of 2.0 and 9.0 if you don't know, and then choose from the other three. The answer is 7.4.
- **Eliminate answers with absolutes.** Most answers are wrong if they contain all inclusive words like always, never, entirely, at no time, absolutely, etc. If you must guess, choose from answers that contain qualifying words such as generally, usually, typically, for the most part, etc.
- **Eliminate choices with little information.** If you must guess between an answer that has a lot of information versus one that has little, choose the one with the most information. A long alternative is usually more correct than a short one.

- **Eliminate the more specific alternative.** When choosing between a general answer and a more specific one, usually the more general alternative is the correct answer.
- **Choose an opposite option.** When two totally opposite answers are given, one of those is likely to be correct. In that case, eliminate all other answers and choose between the two opposites.
- **Do not be fooled by "all of the above."** Here are the rules for dealing with *all the above* and *none of the above* answers: if at least one of the answers is true, then eliminate the answer "none of the above." If at least two of the answers are true then the answer must be "all of the above."
- **Do not change answers.** Students are notorious for changing answers they are not sure of. Usually your first choice is the correct one, so unless you're certain that you made a mistake the first time, don't change your answer.
- **Look for grammatical correctness.** Teachers are typically good at writing questions and answers that are grammatically correct. So, if a question asks for a singular answer, don't choose the plural. For example, serine is "an" Amino Acid, not "an" carbohydrate.

True-False Questions

As easy as they may seem, true-false questions can really be tricky, especially if they're part of a standardized exam. One of the reasons is that teachers who write true-false questions like to include traps for students who don't pay attention to details. It's not that they want to be mean to students; it's that they want to make sure that students know the material. To answer these types of questions, you need to be on the alert for those traps. Here are some suggestions:

- **Watch for extreme qualifiers.** One word can make the difference between a true and false statement. These "all or none" words usually indicate a false answer and include all, always, entirely, every, invariably, never, and none. On the other hand, true statements typically include words like generally, ordinarily, usually, and for the most part.
- **Look for partial false statements.** If any part of a question or statement is false, then the entire statement must be false. For example, in the statement "*The human body consists of more than 60,000 miles of blood vessels, all of them bringing oxygenated blood to cells, tissues and organs.*" This statement may seem true, but it's not since some blood vessels like veins bring deoxygenated blood back to the heart. Another clue was the phrase "all of them," which was a qualifier.
- **Watch for negative words.** These can change the entire meaning of a statement. Here are two examples:
  True: It is *characteristic* for politicians to be talkative.
  False: It is *uncharacteristic* for politicians to be talkative.
  Also, watch out for double negatives that could change the meaning of a statement. So when you see a phrase such as *not unlikely*, scratch it out and make it into *likely*.

- **Guess true if you are not sure.** In most cases, a true-false exam will contain mostly true answers, so you will have a better chance of getting it right. Of course, some teachers know this and will make most answers false, but that's usually not the case.

Short Answer Questions

The two keys to answering short answer questions are quickness and clarity. You must organize your thoughts rapidly, be able to put them in writing, and give explanations and examples to clarify what you're trying to say. Most short answer questions are graded on the overall quality of the response and the thoughtfulness and completeness of the answer. Therefore, knowing the material well is going to help you formulate the answer quickly in your mind. The following are some tips for answering these types of questions in the best way possible:

- **Read the question carefully.** In some cases, short answer questions have several parts. Make sure you read and, if you must, reread the question so that you understand what you're being asked. When you finish answering the question, go back and check to see if you left anything out.
- **Begin with a topic sentence.** You can either restate part of the sentence that you will use to address the question or statement or begin with a key point that will address the rest of your answer. Here's an example:

  Question: During cell division, describe the main differences between mitosis and meiosis.

  Opening sentence: Mitosis and meiosis differ mainly in that mitosis involves cell duplication while in meiosis there is a reduction in the number of chromosomes.
- **Be concise.** By definition, short answers are brief and to the point. There should not be any extra wording that will take away from the main point. So, organize your thoughts, don't ramble or use long sentences, and be specific and detailed. With these types of answers, longer is not always better.
- **Use examples.** When tackling a short answer question, it helps to include an example to illustrate your point. After introducing the key point in your opening sentence and then discussing it, you might add a sentence that begins with *for example, during mitosis the chromosomes . . .*
- **Never skip a question.** First, if you don't know an answer, go on to another question. Even when you're working on another answer, you'll be processing the previous question in your brain and will eventually recall the information. Secondly, even if you don't, the physical act of writing something, even if it's only a few thoughts, will trigger your memory. Besides, there's always partial credit, and most teachers will give you something.

Essay Questions

With emails and texting so common today, many students have a difficult time with essay questions. Their grammar and sentence structure are poor, and they have trouble organizing their thoughts. They spend so much time every day using slang and abbreviations that when it comes to writing a clear, concise, and thoughtful essay, they are at a loss. If you're one of those students, you're going to be at a real disadvantage. Therefore it's very important to learn early on how to write well.

Essay questions can be easier than multiple choice or true-false questions because you have more time to answer them and you can include more information, examples, and illustrations. Also, once you begin writing, it's amazing how quickly your brain will take over and help you sort through the material you've learned. Here are some strategies for answering essay questions:

- **Stop for a moment and think.** If you have studied the material well, you know that it's in your brain. Sometimes closing your eyes and taking a brief pause to think about the question will jar your memory and give you the confidence to start writing.
- **Highlight the key points.** To make sure you understand the question, read it carefully and underline the main point of the question. If the question asks you to address several points, underline each of them so that you don't miss any.
- **Make a brief outline.** Like most students, you probably skip over this step because you think it's a waste of time. In fact, by making a quick outline with key points that you're going to address, you'll be better prepared to answer the question and you'll not forget to include important information. You'll also be better organized and able to write in a clear and concise manner.
- **Organize your paragraphs.** Write a short introduction and then concentrate on the body of your essay. At the end, write a brief conclusion. To maintain clarity, focus on only one key idea in each paragraph, and edit your work when you're done. Don't include opinions unless the question asks for it, and never add irrelevant or extra information just to make your essay longer. That never works.
- **Always include examples and evidence.** This is even more important when answering essay questions than it is when answering short answer questions. If your class lecture notes include illustrations or examples, use those. If not, come up with your own. Examples are a great way to show that you understand the concepts; and as a teacher I'm always impressed when students use good examples to illustrate key points.
- **Use essay key words to answer a question.** Key words are critical in answering an essay question and getting the most points possible. I cannot tell you how many times I've had to take points off a question because a student, who knew the material well enough, did not answer the question like I wanted it answered. Here are the most important keywords to look out for:

  Compare and contrast: To compare is to explain similarities; to contrast is to explain the differences. When a question asks you to compare or contrast something, explain how they're similar or different; don't write a list of their similarities and differences. To prevent doing that, give specific examples. You might write a few sentences about how mitosis and meiosis are different and then add a paragraph starting with: For example: mitosis is a process in which the cell makes an exact copy of itself, whereas in meiosis, the cell is reducing the number of chromosomes in half.

Describe or Discuss: When asked to describe or discuss something, you need to be more detailed and provide a thoughtful, concise, and logical explanation. This is not simply a list of facts. For example, when asked to describe the characteristics of mammals, do not just list the basic characteristics like hair or fur, mammary glands, warm-bloodedness, etc. Describe what fur does and give examples of mammals that survive cold because of fur. Describe how mammary glands function and why they are important to survival.

Interpret: To interpret means to explain something from a graph, chart, figure, or illustration in your own words. Look at the data and think about it for a minute. Once you have analyzed it, explain what you see in writing.

List: When an essay question asks you to include a list, make sure you explain beforehand what the list is. As an example, an essay question might ask you to describe the concept of global warming and list the factors that may be causing it. In this case, spend some time describing what global warming is and then list the factors that may be contributing to it.

Diagram or illustrate: This one is simple and straightforward. When asked to include a diagram, make a drawing and label it. Do not assume the instructor will figure out what you have drawn or that he/she assumes you know what you are drawing. Labels indicate that you know the material.

- **Be neat and use proper grammar.** Even though most instructors will not take off for sloppiness and poor grammar, unless it's an English exam, they may not look at your answer as favorably. However, with the emphasis on reading and writing skills these days, many instructors will take off for grammar. If you want as many points as possible, be neat and construct your sentences in a way that makes sense. After all, it doesn't matter if you know the material if you can't explain it in a way that's readable. There is nothing more frustrating than trying to figure out how to write something when the clock is running.

Math Questions

For many students, math is their hardest subject because they're learning a new language consisting of numbers and constantly expanding formulas. They find that they need to study more for math than for any of their other classes; and if they fall behind in math topics, it's hard to catch up because math concepts and principles build on one another. Probably no other subject requires that you know one concept before going on to the next.

Taking math exams is no different than taking any other exam in that you need to be taking good notes, studying all along, and not cramming the night before. However, being good at math requires a lot of practice working a variety of different problems because you'll be tested on skill rather than on rote memorization. And just like anything else, to get good at a particular skill, you need to practice that skill over and over. The following are some effective strategies for developing those math skills and doing well on any math exam:

- **Do your homework.** Math requires more than study; it requires practice and repetition; and there is no way that you'll do well on exams if you do not work problems outside of class. Use your textbook and any other sources you can find to work a variety of problems. Instructors will often use homework assignments to make up exam questions, and it's a great feeling to see a problem identical to one you've already worked out.
- **Make a crib sheet.** On a single sheet of paper, write down important formulas. Review the sheet every time you study and work homework problems. Before the exam, go over your crib sheet one final time and make sure that you've memorized all the important formulas.
- **Ask questions.** Don't move on to the next concept until you're sure you understand the last one. Remember, all math principles build on each other, so always attend review sessions, and ask your instructor to explain any material that you do not understand.
- **Learn to do word problems.** Word math problems make students panic like no other math problem does. These can be made a lot easier if you've studied the material well and can use the concepts you've learned to solve the problems. No matter what kind of word problem you're asked to solve, there are certain rules to follow. They are:

    1. ***Read the question twice.*** Most students make the mistake of reading a question quickly and then starting to answer it right away. What you want to do instead is read the question once to get an idea of what the problem is about and then reread it to make sure that you understand exactly what you're being asked to do. It also helps to underline details and specific facts necessary to answer the question.
    2. ***Write down the variables.*** Choose letters for your known and unknown variables. For example, if the question tells you that a known radius is 15, write: $R = 15$. If a question gives you an unknown variable you need to find, such as the area of a room, write: Let A = area of the room.
    3. ***Make a drawing.*** After reading and rereading, it may help to draw a figure or a table that you can label. Drawings can add clarity and make a problem more understandable. You might even get partial credit if the instructor sees that you were on the right track.
    4. ***Translate key words.*** One of the biggest stumbling blocks in doing word problems in math is figuring out the equation to use in order to solve the problem. So, to do well on a word problem, you must translate English into the language of symbols and mathematics. The following table illustrates how key

words are identified to determine which mathematical operation to use.

Key Words	Mathematical Operations
increased by, total of, sum, together, more than, combined	Addition
decreased by, less than, minus, difference of, fewer than	Subtraction
multiplied by, the product of, times, of	Multiplication
Per, ratio of, quotient of, percent of, out of	Division
Yields, was, were, is, are, was, were, gives	Equal

- **Write down key formulas.** Unless your instructor allows you to bring a crib sheet to the exam, write down key formulas in the margins or on the back of the exam before you even look at the questions. This will guarantee that you have your formulas handy before the stress of the exam causes you to freeze up.
- **Work the easiest problems first.** Take a quick survey of the exam and pick out the easiest problems. Doing these first will ensure that you have enough time to work on harder problems later. It will also ease anxiety and help build confidence. If you find yourself spending too much time on a single question, skip it and go back to it later.
- **Work neatly.** Careless mistakes translate into lost points; so be neat and show your work in a clean and orderly manner. You'll often get partial credit for a wrong answer if you've written down all the steps. If all you did was make a minor addition or subtraction error, or misplaced a decimal, you'll probably get most of the points anyway.
- **Go back over your work.** At the end of the exam, go back over your work and correct any mistakes or omissions. If you're not sure of your initial answer but cannot decide if another answer is more correct, then leave it alone. Unless you're certain about your correction, the first answer is usually the right one. Besides, students who spend a lot of time dwelling on a question can talk themselves into a wrong answer.

Overcoming Test Anxiety

It's good to be concerned about exams and your grades; it's not good to have text anxiety because that can interfere with your ability to do well on future exams. Students who suffer from text anxiety can be extremely self-critical, and they tend to worry about how grades will affect their future. Instead of feeling challenged by the prospect of success, they become so afraid of failure that they become stressed at the very thought of taking an exam. When they do poorly, it makes them think that they're not the good student they thought they were. They often blame the teacher for their poor performance, which makes correcting the problem even more difficult.

One of the biggest problems with test anxiety is that it directs your attention away from the material you need to learn and away from productive ways to study. You become less organized and less effective in your study habits, which then leads to poor test scores and low grades. This can be very frustrating, especially if it keeps happening in all your courses. Overcoming text anxiety is simple, but it requires that you get in the habit of doing certain things. Here are some effective tips:

- **Space out study.** The worse thing to do is wait until the last minute to study. By spreading out your study sessions over days or weeks, and reviewing several times, you'll feel more prepared and decrease anxiety. The night before the exam, go over the material but don't cram. Rest, exercise, eat well, and get a good night's sleep.
- **Avoid negative students.** Negativism is spread to even good students. If someone is continually negative, it's time to find new study partners who have positive attitudes.
- **Maintain a regular routine during exam week.** Nothing is more disruptive to good study habits and effective learning than starting something new during exam week. So maintain your focus and concentrate on learning rather than on something that will take your mind off schoolwork.
- **Come prepared.** Have a special exam kit that includes pens, pencils, erasers, paper, ruler, calculator, tissues, and, if allowed, a small snack you can quietly munch on.
- **Read directions carefully.** As soon as the test is handed out, read the directions. If there's something you don't understand, ask right away. Never wait until you're well into the exam before asking the instructor for clarification.
- **Write down important information immediately.** As soon as you get the exam, spend the first few minutes writing down formulas, ideas, facts, and key words in the margins or on the back of the exam. Do this before you see the questions. Then, when you start answering questions, refer to your notes. Having the information written down is a great way to ease the anxiety of coming up with answers on the spot.
- **Assess the questions.** Scan the test before you begin to see what types of questions are being asked (multiple choice, essay, matching, etc.) and the number of points they are worth. This way you'll know how to budget your time, which questions are worth the most points, and which ones you will need to spend more time on.
- **Answer the easiest questions first.** This gets you off to a good start and helps build confidence for the remaining questions. Then, when you come to the remaining questions, don't get upset if you come across one you can't answer. Skip it and go on to the next. Your brain will subconsciously process that information and, before long, it will trigger your memory. If you dwell on questions you can't answer, you'll get flustered and will be wasting a lot of time not answering the questions you do know.

Before thinking about medical school, you must first do well in a premedical curriculum. The strategies and techniques in this chapter will boost your learning skills, teach you how to study effectively, and help you do well on the exams you take. The more you condition yourself to be a good learner, the easier it gets. By starting now, you will get in the habit of becoming a lifelong learner that any college or medical school will want.

APPENDIX A

U.S. MEDICAL SCHOOLS

The following is a list of U.S. medical schools. In the most recent admissions data, there were more than 967,000 applications from 52,577 applicants, an average of more than 18 applications per student. 22,981 applicants were accepted to at least one school. For more detailed information and curricula information, see the school's webpage since some of the newer schools have not released any admissions data. Included below are the most recent numbers of in-state and out-of-state applicants, enrollments for both male and female applicants, and in-state matriculant rates. The application deadlines for medical schools are subject to change, but schools always post the latest dates they will accept applications. Always check with your premed advisor and with the medical school for the latest changes in admission requirements and application deadlines.

The percentage of in-state residents interviewed is typically much higher than out-of-state residents. For example, the total percent of applicants interviewed may be 50%, but the percentage of in-state residents interviewed is typically 85% versus 15% for out-of-state residents. The actual numbers of students interviewed from in and out-of-state may be obtained from the AAMC Medical School Admissions Requirements. Consult the latest school catalogues for the most recent tuition, fees, and other expenses. Also included are the eighteen schools that offer financial-based and academic-based free tuition.

ALABAMA

University of Alabama Heersink School of Medicine, Birmingham, AL
In-state applicants: 556; out-of-state applicants: 3,892. First year enrollment: 86 men, 100 women. In-state acceptance rate: 85%.

University of South Alabama Whiddon College of Medicine, Mobile, AL
In-state applicants: 484; out-of-state applicants: 1,102. First year enrollment: 33 men, 45 women. In-state acceptance rate: 92%.

ARIZONA

University of Arizona College of Medicine, Tucson, AZ
In-state applicants: 702; out-of-state applicants: 6,321. First year enrollment: 43 men, 75

women. In-state acceptance rate: 75%.

University of Arizona College of Medicine - Phoenix, Phoenix, AZ
In-state applicants: 700; out-of-state applicants: 5,184. First year enrollment: 62 men, 58 women. In-state acceptance rate: 50%.

ARKANSAS

University of Arkansas College of Medicine, Little Rock, AR
In-state applicants: 319; out-of-state applicants: 2,119. First year enrollment: 78 men, 97 women. In-state acceptance rate: 98%.

CALIFORNIA

California Northstate University College of Medicine, Elk Grove, CA
In-state applicants: 2,490; out-of-state applicants: 1,188. First year enrollment: 58 men, 61 women. In-state acceptance rate: 88%.

Charles R. Drew University of Medicine and Science at UCLA, Los Angeles, CA
In-state applicants: 387; out-of-state applicants: 587. First year enrollment: 25 men, 25 women. In-state acceptance rate: 54%.

Kaiser Permanente Bernard J. Tyson School of Medicine, Pasadena, CA
In-state applicants: 3,873; out-of-state applicants: 3,858. First year enrollment: 103 men, 83 women. In-state acceptance rate: 91%. Tuition-free based on financial need.

Loma Linda University School of Medicine, Loma Linda, CA
In-state applicants: 2,353; out-of-state applicants: 2,784. First year enrollment: 89 men, 87 women. In-state acceptance rate: 52%.

Stanford University School of Medicine, Stanford, CA
In-state applicants: 2,872; out-of-state applicants: 5,965. First year enrollment: 42 men, 47 women. In-state acceptance rate: 33%. Tuition-free based on financial need.

University of California, Davis, School of Medicine, Sacramento, CA
In-state applicants: 5,044; out-of-state applicants: 3,171. First year enrollment: 48 men, 88 women. In-state acceptance rate: 96%.

University of California, Irvine, College of Medicine, Irvine, CA
In-state applicants: 5,026; out-of-state applicants: 2,004. First year enrollment: 40 men, 72 women. In-state acceptance rate: 86%.

University of California David Geffen School of Medicine, Los Angeles, CA
In-state applicants: 6,022; out-of-state applicants: 7,041. First year enrollment: 69 men, 104 women. In-state acceptance rate: 58%. Tuition-free based on academic merit.

University of California, Merced School of Medicine, Merced, CA
In-state applicants: 3,493; out-of-state applicants: 1,325. First year enrollment: 63 men, 66 women. In-state acceptance rate: 98%.

University of California, Riverside, School of Medicine, Riverside, CA
In-state applicants: 4,576; out-of-state applicants: 1,501. First year enrollment: 38 men, 48 women. In-state acceptance rate: 99%.

University of California, San Diego, School of Medicine, San Diego, CA
In-state applicants: 4,889; out-of-state applicants: 3,862. First year enrollment: 46 men, 93 women. In-state acceptance rate: 77%.

University of California, San Francisco, School of Medicine, San Francisco, CA
In-state applicants: 4,193; out-of-state applicants: 4,654. First year enrollment: 64 men, 103 women. In-state acceptance rate: 70%.

University of Southern California Keck School of Medicine, Los Angeles, CA
In-state applicants: 4,358; out-of-state applicants: 4,306. First year enrollment: 81 men, 105 women. In-state acceptance rate: 80%. Tuition-free based on financial need.

COLORADO

University of Colorado School of Medicine, Denver, CO
In-state applicants: 699; out-of-state applicants: 9,152. First year enrollment: 78 men, 102 women. In-state acceptance rate: 43%.

CONNECTICUT

Quinnipiac University Frank Netter School of Medicine, North Haven, CT
In-state applicants: 370; out-of-state applicants: 7,185. First year enrollment: 33 men, 62 women. In-state acceptance rate: 14%.

University of Connecticut School of Medicine, Farmington, CT
In-state applicants: 473; out-of-state applicants: 3,862. First year enrollment: 48 men, 64 women. In-state acceptance rate: 76%.

Yale University School of Medicine, New Haven, CT
In-state applicants: 230; out-of-state applicants: 6,158. First year enrollment: 54 men, 51 women. In-state acceptance rate: 7%.

DISTRICT OF COLUMBIA

George Washington School of Medicine and Health Sciences, Washington, DC
In-state applicants: 642; out-of-state applicants: 15,998. First year enrollment: 86 men, 92 women. In-state acceptance rate: 2%.

Georgetown University School of Medicine, Washington, DC
In-state applicants: 641; out-of-state applicants: 15,954. First year enrollment: 74 men, 126 women. In-state acceptance rate: 3%.

Howard University College of Medicine, Washington, DC
In-state applicants: 423; out-of-state applicants: 8,424. First year enrollment: 59 men, 68

women. In-state acceptance rate: 2%.

FLORIDA

Florida Atlantic University Charles E. Schmidt College of Medicine, Boca Raton, FL
In-state applicants: 2,538; out-of-state applicants: 3,698. First year enrollment: 50 men, 70 women. In-state acceptance rate: 82%.

Florida International University Herbert Wertheim College of Medicine, Miami, FL
In-state applicants: 2,495; out-of-state applicants: 2,177. First year enrollment: 52 men, 70 women. In-state acceptance rate: 81%.

Florida State University College of Medicine, Tallahassee, FL
In-state applicants: 2,661; out-of-state applicants: 4,041. First year enrollment: 40 men, 80 women. In-state acceptance rate: 98%.

Nova Southeastern Patel School of Medicine,
In-state applicants: 2,042; out-of-state applicants: 3,538. First year enrollment: 29 men, 24 women. In-state acceptance rate: 60%.

University of Central Florida College of Medicine, Orlando, FL
In-state applicants: 2,392; out-of-state applicants: 2,560. First year enrollment: 66 men, 54 women. In-state acceptance rate: 63%.

University of Florida College of Medicine, Gainesville, FL
In-state applicants: 2,445; out-of-state applicants: 2,871. First year enrollment: 62 men, 73 women. In-state acceptance rate: 84%.

University of Miami Leonard M. Miller School of Medicine, Miami, FL
In-state applicants: 2,183; out-of-state applicants: 7,923. First year enrollment: 90 men, 111 women. In-state acceptance rate: 47%.

University of South Florida Health Morsani College of Medicine, Tampa, FL
In-state applicants: 2,263; out-of-state applicants: 3,244. First year enrollment: 94 men, 88 women. In-state acceptance rate: 46%.

GEORGIA

Emory University School of Medicine, Atlanta, GA
In-state applicants: 953; out-of-state applicants: 11,929. First year enrollment: 40 men, 99 women. In-state acceptance rate: 40%. Tuition-free based on financial need.

Medical College of Georgia, Augusta, GA
In-state applicants: 1,334; out-of-state applicants: 2,001. First year enrollment: 115 men, 148 women. In-state acceptance rate: 99%.

Mercer University School of Medicine, Macon, GA

In-state applicants: 1,351; out-of-state applicants: 0. First year enrollment: 74 men, 96 women. In-state acceptance rate: 100%.

Morehouse School of Medicine, Atlanta, GA
In-state applicants: 818; out-of-state applicants: 6,174. First year enrollment: 40 men, 70 women. In-state acceptance rate: 68%.

HAWAII

University of Hawaii, John A. Burns School of Medicine, Honolulu, HI
In-state applicants: 219; out-of-state applicants: 2,160. First year enrollment: 24 men, 43 women. In-state acceptance rate: 83%.

ILLINOIS

Carle Illinois College of Medicine, Champaign, IL
In-state applicants: 477; out-of-state applicants: 65. First year enrollment: 2736 men, 11 women. In-state acceptance rate: 14%.

Loyola University Chicago Stritch School of Medicine, Maywood, IL
In-state applicants: 1,392; out-of-state applicants: 10,610. First year enrollment: 56 men, 113 women. In-state acceptance rate: 31%.

Northwestern University Feinberg School of Medicine, Chicago, IL
In-state applicants: 870; out-of-state applicants: 6,966. First year enrollment: 65 men, 80 women. In-state acceptance rate: 28%.

Rosalind Franklin University of Medicine and Science, North Chicago, IL
In-state applicants: 1,268; out-of-state applicants: 8,641. First year enrollment: 94 men, 107 women. In-state acceptance rate: 56%.

Rush Medical College of Rush University Medical Center, Chicago, IL
In-state applicants: 1,295; out-of-state applicants: 10,698. First year enrollment: 67 men, 74 women. In-state acceptance rate: 23%.

Southern Illinois University School of Medicine, Springfield, IL
In-state applicants: 1,035; out-of-state applicants: 90. First year enrollment: 31 men, 49 women. In-state acceptance rate: 100%.

University of Chicago Pritzker School of Medicine, Chicago, IL
In-state applicants: 728; out-of-state applicants: 5,835. First year enrollment: 45 men, 43 women. In-state acceptance rate: 17%.

University of Illinois at Chicago College of Medicine, Chicago, IL
In-state applicants: 1,581; out-of-state applicants: 7,556. First year enrollment: 124 men, 160 women. In-state acceptance rate: 56%.

INDIANA

Indiana University School of Medicine, Indianapolis, IN
In-state applicants: 739; out-of-state applicants: 5,369. First year enrollment: 178 men, 186 women. In-state acceptance rate: 78%.

Indiana University School of Medicine, Evansville, IN
In-state applicants: 438; out-of-state applicants: 2,668. First year enrollment: 103 men, 83 women. In-state acceptance rate: 91%.

IOWA

University of Iowa, Carver College of Medicine, Iowa City, IA
In-state applicants: 295; out-of-state applicants: 3,100. First year enrollment: 79 men, 73 women. In-state acceptance rate: 66%.

KANSAS

University of Kansas School of Medicine, Kansas City, KS
In-state applicants: 444; out-of-state applicants: 2,771. First year enrollment: 112 men, 97 women. In-state acceptance rate: 74%.

KENTUCKY

University of Kentucky College of Medicine, Lexington, KY
In-state applicants: 572; out-of-state applicants: 3,574. First year enrollment: 93 men, 108 women. In-state acceptance rate: 78%.

University of Louisville School of Medicine, Louisville, KY
In-state applicants: 475; out-of-state applicants: 5,113. First year enrollment: 67 men, 95 women. In-state acceptance rate: 73%.

LOUISIANA

Louisiana State University School of Medicine in New Orleans, New Orleans, LA
In-state applicants: 669; out-of-state applicants: 3,222. First year enrollment: 74 men, 120 women. In-state acceptance rate: 91%.

Louisiana State University School of Medicine in Shreveport, Shreveport, LA
In-state applicants: 671; out-of-state applicants: 3,397. First year enrollment: 70 men, 80 women. In-state acceptance rate: 95%.

Tulane University School of Medicine, New Orleans, LA
In-state applicants: 456; out-of-state applicants: 15,252. First year enrollment: 74 men, 116 women. In-state acceptance rate: 24%.

MARYLAND

Johns Hopkins University School of Medicine, Baltimore, MD

In-state applicants: 411; out-of-state applicants: 5,547. First year enrollment: 50 men, 70 women. In-state acceptance rate: 13%.

Uniformed Services University of Health Sciences School of Medicine, Bethesda, MD
In-state applicants: 196; out-of-state applicants: 2,321. First year enrollment: 92 men, 84 women. In-state acceptance rate: 11%. Tuition-free based on future military service.

University of Maryland School of Medicine, Baltimore, MD
In-state applicants: 1,023; out-of-state applicants: 4,661. First year enrollment: 58 men, 88 women. In-state acceptance rate: 81%.

MASSACHUSETTS

Boston University Chobanian Avedisian School of Medicine, Boston, MA
In-state applicants: 909; out-of-state applicants: 9,664. First year enrollment: 64 men, 82 women. In-state acceptance rate: 27%.

Harvard Medical School, Boston, MA
In-state applicants: 639; out-of-state applicants: 7,247. First year enrollment: 69 men, 93 women. In-state acceptance rate: 12%. Tuition-free based on financial need.

Tufts University School of Medicine, Boston, MA
In-state applicants: 1,099; out-of-state applicants: 12,817. First year enrollment: 80 men, 121 women. In-state acceptance rate: 26%.

University of Massachusetts Medical School, Worcester, MA
In-state applicants: 1,090; out-of-state applicants: 4,174. First year enrollment: 55 men, 143 women. In-state acceptance rate: 67%.

MICHIGAN

Central Michigan University College of Medicine, Saginaw, MI
In-state applicants: 1,317; out-of-state applicants: 6,861. First year enrollment: 42 men, 62 women. In-state acceptance rate: 77%.

Michigan State University College of Human Medicine, East Lansing, MI
In-state applicants: 1,552; out-of-state applicants: 5,700. First year enrollment: 82 men, 107 women. In-state acceptance rate: 79%.

Oakland University William Beaumont School of Medicine, Rochester, MI
In-state applicants: 1,364; out-of-state applicants: 6,170. First year enrollment: 48 men, 77 women. In-state acceptance rate: 55%.

University of Michigan Medical School, Ann Arbor, MI
In-state applicants: 1,213; out-of-state applicants: 7,703. First year enrollment: 71 men, 92 women. In-state acceptance rate: 52%. Tuition-free based on academic merit.

Wayne State University School of Medicine, Detroit, MI
In-state applicants: 1,594; out-of-state applicants: 6,455. First year enrollment: 153 men,

151 women. In-state acceptance rate: 62%.

Western Michigan University Homer Stryker M.D. School of Medicine,
In-state applicants: 1,133; out-of-state applicants: 2,971. First year enrollment: 37 men, 47 women. In-state acceptance rate: 39%.

MINNESOTA

Mayo Medical School, Rochester, MN
In-state applicants: 336; out-of-state applicants: 5,167. First year enrollment: 58 men, 50 women. In-state acceptance rate: 9%.

University of Minnesota Medical School, Minneapolis, MN
In-state applicants: 898; out-of-state applicants: 5,089. First year enrollment: 104 men, 134 women. In-state acceptance rate: 83%.

MISSISSIPPI

University of Mississippi School of Medicine, Jackson, MS
In-state applicants: 369; out-of-state applicants: 19. First year enrollment: 74 men, 91 women. In-state acceptance rate: 100%.

MISSOURI

Saint Louis University School of Medicine, St. Louis, MO
In-state applicants: 407; out-of-state applicants: 5,670. First year enrollment: 76 men, 102 women. In-state acceptance rate: 34%.

University of Missouri-Columbia School of Medicine, Columbia, MO
In-state applicants: 548; out-of-state applicants: 2,151. First year enrollment: 45 men, 83 women. In-state acceptance rate: 84%.

University of Missouri-Kansas City School of Medicine, Kansas City, MO
In-state applicants: 345; out-of-state applicants: 1,550. First year enrollment: 47 men, 89 women. In-state acceptance rate: 64%.

Washington University in St. Louis School of Medicine, St. Louis, MO
In-state applicants: 268; out-of-state applicants: 5,433. First year enrollment: 62 men, 62 women. In-state acceptance rate: 6%. Tuition-free based on financial need.

NEBRASKA

Creighton University School of Medicine, Omaha, NE
In-state applicants: 156; out-of-state applicants: 6,085. First year enrollment: 127 men, 126 women. In-state acceptance rate: 4%.

University of Nebraska College of Medicine, Omaha, NE
In-state applicants: 261; out-of-state applicants: 1,812. First year enrollment: 58 men, 74

women. In-state acceptance rate: 80%.

NEVADA

University of Nevada Kerkorian School of Medicine, Las Vegas, NV
In-state applicants: 268; out-of-state applicants: 1,292. First year enrollment: 30 men, 36 women. In-state acceptance rate: 73%.

University of Nevada School of Medicine, Reno, NV
In-state applicants: 295; out-of-state applicants: 1,369. First year enrollment: 31 men, 39 women. In-state acceptance rate: 83%.

NEW HAMPSHIRE

Dartmouth University Geisel School of Medicine, Hanover, NH
In-state applicants: 682; out-of-state applicants: 8,453. First year enrollment: 45 men, 47 women. In-state acceptance rate: 3%.

NEW JERSEY

Cooper Medical School of Rowan University, Camden, NJ
In-state applicants: 1,262; out-of-state applicants: 3,295. First year enrollment: 54 men, 58 women. In-state acceptance rate: 78%.

Hackensack Meridian School of Medicine, Nutley, NJ
In-state applicants: 1,235; out-of-state applicants: 4,941. First year enrollment: 83 men, 79 women. In-state acceptance rate: 52%.

Rutgers New Jersey Medical School, Newark, NJ
In-state applicants: 1,506; out-of-state applicants: 4,353. First year enrollment: 76 men, 97 women. In-state acceptance rate: 84%.

Rutgers Robert Wood Johnson Medical School, Piscataway, NJ
In-state applicants: 1,485; out-of-state applicants: 4,315. First year enrollment: 54 men, 111 women. In-state acceptance rate: 89%

NEW MEXICO

University of New Mexico School of Medicine, Albuquerque, NM
In-state applicants: 195; out-of-state applicants: 1,534. First year enrollment: 45 men, 50 women. In-state acceptance rate: 94%.

NEW YORK

Albany Medical College, Albany, NY
In-state applicants: 2,055; out-of-state applicants: 11,203. First year enrollment: 64 men, 79 women. In-state acceptance rate: 29%.

Albert Einstein College of Medicine of Yeshiva University, Bronx, NY
In-state applicants: 1,793; out-of-state applicants: 7,219. First year enrollment: 76 men, 107 women. In-state acceptance rate: 49%. Tuition-free for all incoming students.

Columbia University College of Physicians and Surgeons, New York, NY
In-state applicants: 1,109; out-of-state applicants: 6,094. First year enrollment: 67 men, 71 women. In-state acceptance rate: 17%. Tuition-free based on financial need.

Donald and Barbara Zucker School of Medicine at Hofstra/Northwell, Hempstead, NY
In-state applicants: 1,561; out-of-state applicants: 3,473. First year enrollment: 50 men, 49 women. In-state acceptance rate: 65%.

Icahn School of Medicine at Mount Sinai, New York, NY
In-state applicants: 1,481; out-of-state applicants: 7,033. First year enrollment: 55 men, 65 women. In-state acceptance rate: 27%. Tuition-free based on financial need.

New York Medical College, Valhalla, NY
In-state applicants: 2,123; out-of-state applicants: 8,439. First year enrollment: 98 men, 121 women. In-state acceptance rate: 58%.

NYU Grossman School of Medicine, New York, NY
In-state applicants: 1,172; out-of-state applicants: 6,909. First year enrollment: 47 men, 53 women. In-state acceptance rate: 7%. Tuition-free based on financial need.

NYU Grossman Long Island School of Medicine, Mineola, NY
In-state applicants: 1,092; out-of-state applicants: 2,953. First year enrollment: 10 men, 14 women. In-state acceptance rate: 50%.

SUNY Downstate Medical Center College of Medicine, Brooklyn, NY
In-state applicants: 2,490; out-of-state applicants: 4,519. First year enrollment: 92 men, 113 women. In-state acceptance rate: 86%.

SUNY Upstate Norton College of Medicine, Syracuse, NY
In-state applicants: 2,220; out-of-state applicants: 3,401. First year enrollment: 67 men, 107 women. In-state acceptance rate: 79%.

Stony Brook University Renaissance School of Medicine, Stony Brook, NY
In-state applicants: 2,067; out-of-state applicants: 3,402. First year enrollment: 63 men, 73 women. In-state acceptance rate: 77%.

University at Buffalo Jacobs School of Medicine, Buffalo, NY
In-state applicants: 2,157; out-of-state applicants: 23,918. First year enrollment: 71 men, 112 women. In-state acceptance rate: 91%.

University of Rochester School of Medicine and Dentistry, Rochester, NY
In-state applicants: 1,345; out-of-state applicants: 4,854. First year enrollment: 52 men, 52 women. In-state acceptance rate: 26%.

Weill Cornell Medical College of Cornell University, New York, NY

In-state applicants: 1,264; out-of-state applicants: 5,957. First year enrollment: 57 men, 49 women. In-state acceptance rate: 30%. Tuition-free based on financial need.

NORTH CAROLINA

Duke University School of Medicine, Durham, NY
In-state applicants: 658; out-of-state applicants: 7,773. First year enrollment: 35 men, 83 women. In-state acceptance rate: 14%. Tuition-free based on academic merit.

East Carolina University Brody School of Medicine, Greenville, NC
In-state applicants: 1,092; out-of-state applicants: 33. First year enrollment: 35 men, 55 women. In-state acceptance rate: 100%.

University of North Carolina School of Medicine, Chapel Hill, NC
In-state applicants: 1,080; out-of-state applicants: 4,728. First year enrollment: 82 men, 122 women. In-state acceptance rate: 88%.

Wake Forest Baptist Medical Center School of Medicine, Winston-Salem, NC
In-state applicants: 917; out-of-state applicants: 11,149. First year enrollment: 55 men, 90 women. In-state acceptance rate: 39%.

NORTH DAKOTA

University of North Dakota School of Medicine and Health Sciences, Grand Forks, ND
In-state applicants: 107; out-of-state applicants: 1,543. First year enrollment: 37 men, 37 women. In-state acceptance rate: 49%.

OHIO

Case Western Reserve University School of Medicine, Cleveland, OH
In-state applicants: 750; out-of-state applicants: 7,865. First year enrollment: 101 men, 111 women. In-state acceptance rate: 18%. Tuition-free based on financial need.

Northeast Ohio Medical University College of Medicine, Rootstown, OH
In-state applicants: 955; out-of-state applicants: 3,704. First year enrollment: 90 men, 84 women. In-state acceptance rate: 83%.

Ohio State University College of Medicine, Columbus, OH
In-state applicants: 1,135; out-of-state applicants: 6,094. First year enrollment: 90 men, 108 women. In-state acceptance rate: 55%.

University of Cincinnati College of Medicine, Cincinnati, OH
In-state applicants: 1,082; out-of-state applicants: 5,099. First year enrollment: 83 men, 94 women. In-state acceptance rate: 57%.

University of Toledo College of Medicine, Toledo, OH
In-state applicants: 1,113; out-of-state applicants: 4,453. First year enrollment: 76 men, 98 women. In-state acceptance rate: 64%.

Wright State University Boonshoft School of Medicine, Dayton, OH
In-state applicants: 1,067; out-of-state applicants: 5,212. First year enrollment: 77 men, 49 women. In-state acceptance rate: 80%.

OKLAHOMA

University of Oklahoma College of Medicine, Oklahoma City, OK
In-state applicants: 329; out-of-state applicants: 1,894 First year enrollment: 99 men, 77 women. In-state acceptance rate: 91%.

OREGON

Oregon Health & Science University School of Medicine, Portland, OR
In-state applicants: 447; out-of-state applicants: 5,844. First year enrollment: 59 men, 89 women. In-state acceptance rate: 72%.

PENNSYLVANIA

Geisinger Commonwealth Medical College, Scranton, PA
In-state applicants: 862; out-of-state applicants: 4,392. First year enrollment: 52 men, 62 women. In-state acceptance rate: 65%.

Drexel University College of Medicine, Philadelphia, PA
In-state applicants: 1,078; out-of-state applicants: 14,769. First year enrollment: 132 men, 172 women. In-state acceptance rate: 33%.

Penn State College of Medicine, Hershey, PA
In-state applicants: 1,052; out-of-state applicants: 10,021. First year enrollment: 50 men, 95 women. In-state acceptance rate: 31%.

Temple University Katz School of Medicine, Philadelphia, PA
In-state applicants: 1,070; out-of-state applicants: 12,302. First year enrollment: 95 men, 126 women. In-state acceptance rate: 38%.

Thomas Jefferson University Sidney Kimmel Medical College, Philadelphia, PA
In-state applicants: 1,027; out-of-state applicants: 9,894. First year enrollment: 126 men, 144 women. In-state acceptance rate: 29%.

University of Pennsylvania Perelman School of Medicine, Philadelphia, PA
In-state applicants: 505; out-of-state applicants: 5,512. First year enrollment: 75 men, 81 women. In-state acceptance rate: 12%. Tuition-free based on academic merit.

University of Pittsburgh School of Medicine, Pittsburgh, PA
In-state applicants: 861; out-of-state applicants: 7,921. First year enrollment: 68 men, 80 women. In-state acceptance rate: 38%.

PUERTO RICO

Ponce Health Sciences University School of Medicine, Ponce, PR
In-state applicants: 516; out-of-state applicants: 1,339. First year enrollment: 86 men, 93 women. In-state acceptance rate: 65%.

San Juan Bautista School of Medicine, San Juan, PR
In-state applicants: 346; out-of-state applicants: 814. First year enrollment: 23 men, 41 women. In-state acceptance rate: 47%.

Universidad Central del Caribe School of Medicine, Bayamon, PR
In-state applicants: 341; out-of-state applicants: 474. First year enrollment: 29 men, 48 women. In-state acceptance rate: 86%.

University of Puerto Rico School of Medicine, San Juan, PR
In-state applicants: 309; out-of-state applicants: 425. First year enrollment: 44 men, 58 women. In-state acceptance rate: 98%.

RHODE ISLAND

Brown University Warren Alpert School of Medicine, Providence, RI
In-state applicants: 89; out-of-state applicants: 8,784. First year enrollment: 58 men, 86 women. In-state acceptance rate: 11%.

SOUTH CAROLINA

Medical University of South Carolina College of Medicine, Charleston, SC
In-state applicants: 556; out-of-state applicants: 3,124. First year enrollment: 70 men, 101 women. In-state acceptance rate: 91%.

University of South Carolina - Columbia School of Medicine, Columbia, SC
In-state applicants: 489; out-of-state applicants: 2,369. First year enrollment: 44 men, 56 women. In-state acceptance rate: 75%.

University of South Carolina - Greenville School of Medicine, Greenville, SC
In-state applicants: 518; out-of-state applicants: 3,869. First year enrollment: 29 men, 41 women. In-state acceptance rate: 70%.

SOUTH DAKOTA

University of South Dakota Sanford School of Medicine, Sioux Falls, SD
In-state applicants: 126; out-of-state applicants: 991. First year enrollment: 36 men, 35 women. In-state acceptance rate: 73%.

TENNESSEE

East Tennessee State University Quillen College of Medicine, Johnson City, TN
In-state applicants: 571; out-of-state applicants: 3,394. First year enrollment: 37 men, 39 women. In-state acceptance rate: 82%.

Meharry Medical College School of Medicine, Nashville, TN
In-state applicants: 323; out-of-state applicants: 7,197. First year enrollment: 49 men, 67 women. In-state acceptance rate: 18%.

Thomas F. Frist, Jr. College of Medicine at Belmont University, Nashville, TN
In-state applicants: 438; out-of-state applicants: 2,668. First year enrollment: 103 men, 83 women. In-state acceptance rate: 91%.

University of Tennessee Health Science Center College of Medicine, Memphis, TN
In-state applicants: 637; out-of-state applicants: 1,965. First year enrollment: 86 men, 87 women. In-state acceptance rate: 90%.

Vanderbilt University School of Medicine, Nashville, TN
In-state applicants: 294; out-of-state applicants: 6,243. First year enrollment: 45 men, 50 women. In-state acceptance rate: 11%. Tuition-free based on academic merit.

TEXAS

Anne Burnett Marion School of Medicine at TCU, Fort Worth, TX
In-state applicants: 1,271; out-of-state applicants: 5,086. First year enrollment: 27 men, 33 women. In-state acceptance rate: 25%.

Baylor College of Medicine, Houston, TX
In-state applicants: 3,984; out-of-state applicants: 1,588. First year enrollment: 109 men, 1017 women. In-state acceptance rate: 83%.

Texas A&M Health Science Center College of Medicine, College Station, TX
In-state applicants: 4,272; out-of-state applicants: 1,319. First year enrollment: 102 men, 97 women. In-state acceptance rate: 86%.

Texas Tech University Health Sciences Center School of Medicine, Lubbock, TX
In-state applicants: 4,065; out-of-state applicants: 904. First year enrollment: 94 men, 87 women. In-state acceptance rate: 90%.

Texas Tech University Paul L. Foster School of Medicine, El Paso, TX
In-state applicants: 3,732; out-of-state applicants: 819. First year enrollment: 66 men, 58 women. In-state acceptance rate: 94%.

University of Houston Tilman J. Fertitta Family College of Medicine, Houston, TX
In-state applicants: 3,968; out-of-state applicants: 925. First year enrollment: 20 men, 40 women. In-state acceptance rate: 97%.

University of Texas at Austin Dell Medical School, Austin, TX
In-state applicants: 4,163; out-of-state applicants: 1,120. First year enrollment: 21 men, 29 women. In-state acceptance rate: 90%.

University of Texas at Tyler School of Medicine, Tyler, TX
In-state applicants: 3,181; out-of-state applicants: 575. First year enrollment: 10 men, 30

women. In-state acceptance rate: 98%.

University of Texas Medical Branch Sealy School of Medicine, Galveston, TX
In-state applicants: 4,185; out-of-state applicants: 963. First year enrollment: 108 men, 120 women. In-state acceptance rate: 94%.

University of Texas McGovern Medical School at Houston, Houston, TX
In-state applicants: 4,305; out-of-state applicants: 1,344. First year enrollment: 109 men, 1131 women. In-state acceptance rate: 95%.

University of Texas Rio Grande Valley School of Medicine, Brownsville, TX
In-state applicants: 3,719; out-of-state applicants: 789. First year enrollment: 22 men, 31 women. In-state acceptance rate: 93%.

University of Texas School of Medicine at San Antonio, San Antonio, TX
In-state applicants: 4,206; out-of-state applicants: 1,172. First year enrollment: 119 men, 112 women. In-state acceptance rate: 88%.

University of Texas Southwestern Medical School, Dallas, TX
In-state applicants: 4,156; out-of-state applicants: 1,371. First year enrollment: 108 men, 121 women. In-state acceptance rate: 87%.

UTAH

University of Utah Eccles School of Medicine, Salt Lake City, UT
In-state applicants: 519; out-of-state applicants: 2,516. First year enrollment: 63 men, 62 women. In-state acceptance rate: 73%.

VERMONT

University of Vermont Larner College of Medicine, Burlington, VT
In-state applicants: 857; out-of-state applicants: 8,483. First year enrollment: 61 men, 56 women. In-state acceptance rate: 27%.

VIRGINIA

Eastern Virginia Medical School, Norfolk, VA
In-state applicants: 1,119; out-of-state applicants: 6,067. First year enrollment: 72 men, 79 women. In-state acceptance rate: 50%.

Virginia Commonwealth University School of Medicine, Richmond, VA
In-state applicants: 1,183; out-of-state applicants: 5,857. First year enrollment: 79 men, 104 women. In-state acceptance rate: 54%.

Virginia Tech Carilion School of Medicine, Roanoke, VA
In-state applicants: 841; out-of-state applicants: 5,343. First year enrollment: 24 men, 24 women. In-state acceptance rate: 16%.

University of Virginia School of Medicine, Charlottesville, VA

In-state applicants: 914; out-of-state applicants: 4,765. First year enrollment: 74 men, 84 women. In-state acceptance rate: 46%.

WASHINGTON

University of Washington School of Medicine, Seattle, WA
In-state applicants: 947; out-of-state applicants: 6,070. First year enrollment: 105 men, 163 women. In-state acceptance rate: 54%.

Washington State University Elson S. Floyd School of Medicine, Spokane, WA
In-state applicants: 830; out-of-state applicants: 784. First year enrollment: 19 men, 61 women. In-state acceptance rate: 89%.

WEST VIRGINIA

Marshall University Joan C. Edwards School of Medicine, Huntington, WV
In-state applicants: 160 out-of-state applicants: 1,681. First year enrollment: 38 men, 34 women. In-state acceptance rate: 57%.

West Virginia University School of Medicine, Morgantown, WV
In-state applicants: 193; out-of-state applicants: 5,030. First year enrollment: 56 men, 56 women. In-state acceptance rate: 70%.

WISCONSIN

Medical College of Wisconsin, Milwaukee, WI
In-state applicants: 690; out-of-state applicants: 8,899. First year enrollment: 116 men, 148 women. In-state acceptance rate: 52%.

University of Wisconsin School of Medicine and Public Health, Madison, WI
In-state applicants: 664; out-of-state applicants: 5,720. First year enrollment: 72 men, 98 women. In-state acceptance rate: 68%.

APPENDIX B

U.S. COLLEGES OF OSTEOPATHIC MEDICINE

Osteopathic physicians (D.O.s) are licensed to practice medicine and surgery in all 50 states and are recognized in sixty other countries, including all Canadian provinces. Techniques of osteopathy rely on holistic treatments such as the manipulation of joints and bones to diagnose and treat illness. Students who want to practice medicine using a more holistic approach may want to consider an osteopathic college. The following is a list of the accredited colleges of osteopathic medicine in the United States.

Alabama College of Osteopathic Medicine, Dothan Al

A.T. Still University of Health Sciences, Kirksville, MO

A.T. Still University of Health Sciences, Mesa, AZ

Arizona College of Osteopathic Medicine, Glendale, AZ

Arkansas College of Osteopathic Medicine, Fort Smith, AR

Burrell College of Osteopathic Medicine New Mexico State University, Las Cruces, NM

California Health Sciences University College of Osteopathic Medicine, Clovis, CA

Campbell University School of Osteopathic Medicine, Lillington, NC

Chicago College of Osteopathic Medicine, Downers Grove, IL

Des Moines University College of Osteopathic Medicine, Des Moines, IA

Edward Via College of Osteopathic Medicine - Carolinas Campus, Auburn, AL

Edward Via College of Osteopathic Medicine - Virginia Campus, Blacksburg, VA

Edward Via College of Osteopathic Medicine - Virginia Campus, Monroe, LA

Edward Via College of Osteopathic Medicine - Virginia Campus, Spartanburg, SC

Georgia Campus Philadelphia College of Osteopathic Medicine, Suwanee, GA

Idaho College of Osteopathic Medicine, Meridian, ID

Kansas City University of Medicine and Biosciences College of Osteopathic Medicine, Kansas City, MO

Kirksville College of Osteopathic Medicine, Kirksville, MO

Lake Erie College of Osteopathic Medicine, Erie, PA

Lake Erie College of Osteopathic Medicine, Bradenton Campus, Bradenton, FL

Liberty University College of Osteopathic Medicine, Lynchburg, VA

Lincoln Memorial University DeBusk College of Osteopathic Medicine, Harrogate, TN

Marian University College of Osteopathic Medicine, Indianapolis, IN

Michigan State University College of Osteopathic Medicine, East Lansing, MI

New York Institute of Technology College of Osteopathic Medicine, Old Westbury, NY

Nova Southeastern University College of Osteopathic Medicine, Fort Lauderdale, FL

Ohio University Heritage College of Osteopathic Medicine, Athens, OH

Oklahoma State University Center for Health Sciences

College of Osteopathic Medicine, Tulsa, OK

Pacific Northwest University of Health Sciences College of Osteopathic Medicine, Yakima, WA

Philadelphia College of Osteopathic Medicine, Philadelphia, PA

Rocky Vista University College of Osteopathic Medicine, Parker, CO

Rowan University School of Osteopathic Medicine, Stratford, NJ

Sam Houston State University College of Osteopathic Medicine, Conroe, TX

Texas College of Osteopathic Medicine, Fort Worth, TX

Touro College of Osteopathic Medicine, New York, NY

Touro University College of Osteopathic Medicine, Vallejo, CA

Touro University Nevada College of Osteopathic Medicine, Henderson, NV

University of the Incarnate Word School of Osteopathic Medicine, San Antonio, TX

University of New England College of Osteopathic Medicine, Biddeford, ME

University of Pikeville Kentucky College of Osteopathic Medicine, Pikeville, KY

West Virginia School of Osteopathic Medicine, Lewisburg, WV

Western University of Health Sciences College of Osteopathic Medicine of the Pacific, Pomona, CA

William Carey University College of Osteopathic Medicine, Hattiesburg, MS

Appendix C

CHECKLIST FOR THE ADMISSIONS PROCESS

- ☐ Freshman year: visit regularly with your premedical advisor and discuss career plans.
- ☐ Outline a 4-year curriculum that includes all the premed requirements, as well as a broad range of electives that will make you a better candidate.
- ☐ Become involved in school and community activities as soon as possible, beginning during your freshman year, and strive for leadership positions.
- ☐ Sophomore year: continue volunteer work in a healthcare setting or by shadowing a physician.
- ☐ Fall, junior year: begin studying for the MCAT.
- ☐ Fall, junior year: register for the MCAT.
- ☐ Spring, junior year: take the MCAT.
- ☐ Spring, junior year: request letters of recommendation.
- ☐ Spring, junior year: begin working on the AMCAS application.
- ☐ Spring, junior year: request a copy of your transcripts.
- ☐ Fall, senior year: submit the AMCAS application by the required deadlines (August through December).
- ☐ Senior year: complete all college degree requirements.
- ☐ Senior year: prepare for medical school interviews.

APPENDIX D

CHECKLIST FOR APPLICATION DEADLINES

Activity	Deadline
Register for the MCAT	
Submit Applications (Names of Schools)	

Appendix E

SUMMARY OF EXTRACURRICULAR ACTIVITIES

School Activities	Dates	Description
Volunteer Work	**Dates**	**Description**
Employment	**Dates**	**Description**
Academic Awards	**Dates**	**Description**

Appendix F

ADMISSIONS SELECTION CRITERIA

The following are admissions selection criteria based on AAMC interviews with admission committee members. Results are based on a scale of what committee members considered the most important criteria to the least important criteria for selecting students.

Most Important	• Cumulative GPA in science and math • MCAT scores • Overall GPA • Selectivity and competitiveness of undergraduate institution • Letters of recommendation • Personal statement, interview assessment • Healthcare experience • Volunteer experience, leadership positions held
Somewhat Important	• Cumulative non-science/math GPA • On schedule to meet premedical coursework • Research experience in private sector • Experience with diverse populations • Family circumstances • Work or athletic scholarship obligations • First-generation college student • Race/ethnicity/socioeconomic status
Least Important	• Completion of non-science coursework • Job in non-medical setting • Research experience in the public sector • Multilingual • Gender

INDEX

ABOUT THE AUTHOR

Dr. Andrew Goliszek received a Ph.D. in Physiology and Endocrinology from Utah State University. He was a research associate at Wake Forest University School of Medicine in both the department of Physiology and Pharmacology and the department of Medicine. Following that, he was Associate Professor of Biology and Human Anatomy & Physiology at North Carolina A&T State University and is the author of numerous articles and books. He has been a premed advisor, research mentor, principal investigator and coinvestigator on several NIH biomedical grants, and was the recipient of the prestigious College of Arts & Sciences Faculty of the Year Award for excellence in teaching, research, and student advising.

Made in the USA
Monee, IL
05 November 2026

67811471R00164